Thieme

Atlas of Ultrasound and Anatomy

Facial Rejuvenation

Steven F. Weiner, MD
Facial Plastic Surgeon and Founder
Aesthetic Clinique
Santa Rosa Beach, Florida, USA

Christopher C. Surek, DO, FACS
Assistant Professor of Anatomy
Department of Anatomy
Kansas City University;
Clinical Assistant Professor
Department of Plastic Surgery
University of Kansas Medical Center;
Board Certified Plastic Surgeon
Private Practice
Surek Plastic Surgery
Kansas City, Missouri, USA

Illustrations by Dr. Levent Efe, CMI

162 Illustrations

Thieme
New York • Stuttgart • Delhi • Rio de Janeiro

Library of Congress Cataloging-in-Publication Data is available from the publisher.

Important note: Medicine is an ever-changing science undergoing continual development. Research and clinical experience are continually expanding our knowledge, in particular our knowledge of proper treatment and drug therapy. Insofar as this book mentions any dosage or application, readers may rest assured that the authors, editors, and publishers have made every effort to ensure that such references are in accordance with **the state of knowledge at the time of production of the book.**

Nevertheless, this does not involve, imply, or express any guarantee or responsibility on the part of the publishers in respect to any dosage instructions and forms of applications stated in the book. **Every user is requested to examine carefully** the manufacturers' leaflets accompanying each drug and to check, if necessary, in consultation with a physician or specialist, whether the dosage schedules mentioned therein or the contraindications stated by the manufacturers differ from the statements made in the present book. Such examination is particularly important with drugs that are either rarely used or have been newly released on the market. Every dosage schedule or every form of application used is entirely at the user's own risk and responsibility. The authors and publishers request every user to report to the publishers any discrepancies or inaccuracies noticed. If errors in this work are found after publication, errata will be posted at www.thieme.com on the product description page.

Some of the product names, patents, and registered designs referred to in this book are in fact registered trademarks or proprietary names even though specific reference to this fact is not always made in the text. Therefore, the appearance of a name without designation as proprietary is not to be construed as a representation by the publisher that it is in the public domain.

Thieme addresses people of all gender identities equally. We encourage our authors to use gender-neutral or gender-equal expressions wherever the context allows.

Thieme Publishers New York
333 Seventh Avenue, 18th Floor
New York, NY 10001, USA
www.thieme.com
+1 800 782 3488, customerservice@thieme.com

Illustrations: © Dr. Levent Efe, CMI
Cover design: © Thieme
Cover image source: © Dr. Levent Efe, CMI/Thieme
Typesetting by TNQ Tech Private Limited, India

Printed in USA by King Printing Co., Inc. 5 4 3 2

DOI: 10.1055/b000001071

ISBN: 978-1-68420-496-0

Also available as an e-book:
eISBN (PDF): 978-1-68420-497-7
eISBN (epub): 978-1-63853-716-8

I dedicate this book to my family. My wife Sandy has been my biggest supporter and cheerleader. I thank my children, Alex and Sydney, who allowed me to practice ultrasound for countless hours during the Covid lockdown. I want to especially thank Dr. Leonie Schelke, who has been my mentor and colleague during my ultrasound journey. I hope readers are inspired to adopt ultrasound and their injections are safer and more precise because of this text.

Steven F. Weiner

I dedicate this book to my family. My wife Krystle Surek and my children Arden Surek and Sutton Surek. They continue to support my passion for education and teaching and my love for this field. I also want to thank all of my mentors over the past several years. Without their guidance, instruction, and support, I would not be the surgeon, injector, and educator that I am today. And lastly, I dedicate this book to you…the reader...we are all in this together, and we must continue to educate ourselves, each other, and our patients. I encourage all of us to never stop learning and always strive for safe, ethical, and consistent results for our patients.

Christopher C. Surek

Contents

Preface

Ultrasonography of the face has become an invaluable addition to the aesthetic industry. Its roots date back to Dr. Philippe Katz (France) who started dermatology ultrasound in 1998 and wrote the first paper in 2000 on using polylactic acid in HIV positive patients where facial ultrasound was incorporated. Other early innovators (2011) were the Amsterdam group of physicians (later known as the Cutaneous group) consisting of Dr. Leonie Schelke, Dr. Peter Velthuis, and then later Dr. Tom Decates. It is this group which has spearheaded the research and education for the use of ultrasound in aesthetic injections and filler complication management. There have been global contributions to ultrasound including Korean experts, Dr. Hyoung Jin Moon, Dr. Ji Soo Kim, and Dr. Hee-Jin Kim, and South American experts, Dr. Ximena Wortsman (2001) and Dr. Rosa Sigrist.

When asked by Dr. Surek to coauthor his next textbook on anatomy for the injector highlighting ultrasound, I was honored and eager to share my knowledge of this burgeoning field. My goal is to show pertinent anatomy for the injector using ultrasound. There is a huge variation of vascular anatomy in patients seeking treatments. This text will show the most common anatomy found in our patients and will further discuss some of the most common variants. It is my belief that having a sound background in anatomy is a prerequisite for understanding ultrasound imaging. That is why combining both detailed medical illustrations and ultrasound images makes sense, and this is the first textbook to include such a comprehensive analysis of facial anatomic relationships.

Unfortunately, still imaging does not do justice to ultrasound. We encourage injectors to practice diligently and appreciate the benefit of real-time video and imaging when assessing their patients. In addition, to maintain focus of this textbook on anatomy, the other benefits of using ultrasound to help analyze and mitigate filler complications were purposely not included.

This textbook is the culmination of hundreds of cadaver dissections, extensive literature reviews, and countless ultrasound images. We try to transfer our wealth of knowledge we have garnered from our decades of surgical and injection experience. The field of facial ultrasound is still very young but growing rapidly. There will undoubtedly be new discoveries, and technologies, including artificial intelligence (AI), emerging in the next couple of years that will drive further adoption by decreasing the learning curve and helping the novice decipher the "70 shades of gray."

Steven F. Weiner, MD

Over the past 12 years, I have been fortunate to research, publish, and educate on facial anatomy specific to injectors, including but not limited to countless dissection hours in the lab with over 500+ cadaver head dissections to date. I have also been involved in many collaborations in evidence-based research, and teaching and speaking at conferences/courses nationally and internationally. Countless mentors and colleagues have guided me and traveled with me on this quest. I am extremely grateful for all of their support and mentorship. This book is a careful summation of what I have learned and discovered along the way.

Anatomy for the filler and neurotoxin injector is inherently unique compared to the anatomy for the facial surgeon or the academic anatomist. It does not necessarily mean that the anatomy is different, it means how one views and uses the anatomy in surgery versus injections is unique. For example, in facelift surgery we often release cheek-retaining ligaments to facilitate flap movement, whereas in filler injection we may use the ligaments as boundaries to build between when restoring or enhancing cheek contour in our patients. In blepharoplasty surgery, often the orbital retaining ligament (ORL) and tear trough ligament (TTL) are released to allow soft tissue repositioning, whereas in filler injection we often rely on the stability and location of these ligaments for boundary support and/or possible volume augmentation in tear trough treatments.

The bottom line is an injector is reliant on a high yield understanding of the clinically relevant anatomy for facial navigation, which impacts patient outcomes and avoids unwanted complications. Until the recent introduction of ultrasound into the medical aesthetics space, soft tissue filler and neurotoxin injection relied on the injector's experience and ability to navigate the face without direct vision of the deeper structures.

With the use of ultrasound in this field, it now provides a new wave of visualization of facial anatomy in our patients.

Ultrasound has become a paramount part of my nonsurgical aesthetics practice. I firmly believe it gives injectors the ability to assess for anatomical variation, assess suboptimal outcomes, treat complications, and possibly provide real time–guided injections. Therefore, Dr. Steve Weiner and I decided to collaborate on an anatomically centered ultrasound atlas, outlining the clinically relevant anatomy for the injector throughout the face coupled with step-by-step guidance for utilizing ultrasound as a facial injector.

In this text, we encourage readers to immerse themselves in the beautiful and intricate three-dimensional architecture of the face, as if they are traveling through an immersive art exhibition. We take you on a journey through key aesthetic subunits, highlighting the different facial layers and the symphony of structures that exist within them. We have taken great care to focus on the high yield anatomical structures and equip the injectors with the necessary knowledge to navigate to their target and avoid undesired outcomes.

Lastly, I encourage all injectors regardless of their level of training or experience to always maintain a healthy fear of the anatomy and to continue to educate themselves throughout their career. Steve and I are hopeful that this book will serve as another resource among many that injectors can utilize to enhance and sharpen their skill set as facial injectors.

Christopher C. Surek, DO, FACS

Chapter 1

A Three-Dimensional Approach to Facial Anatomy for the Injector

1

1 A Three-Dimensional Approach to Facial Anatomy for the Injector

Abstract
Facial anatomy for the injector is predicated upon a strong understanding of the three-dimensional architecture of the face. This chapter will describe the concentric layers of the face as well as the symphony of structures in the face that can be utilized by the injector to optimize outcomes.

Keywords: Superficial musculoaponeurotic system (SMAS), retaining ligaments, potential spaces, facial fat compartments

1.1 Facial Skeleton

Anatomy for the facial injector is unique and complex. It is paramount that the injector has a comprehensive understanding of the three-dimensional architecture of the face. The authors urge injectors to consider the superficial musculoaponeurotic system (SMAS) as a depth gauge to assist in navigating from superficial to deep and vice versa during clinical injection.

Simplistically, the face has five concentric layers (▸ Fig. 1.1, ▸ Fig. 1.2, ▸ Fig. 1.3, ▸ Fig. 1.4).

- **Layer 1** is the facial skeleton and periosteum.
  - Facial skeleton loses bone mineral density with age resulting in morphological changes.
- **Layer 2** is the "sub-SMAS" plane.
  - It contains deep fat compartments, potential spaces, and the origins of the "true" osseocutaneous retaining ligaments.
- **Layer 3** is the SMAS layer.
- **Layer 4** is the "supra-SMAS" layer.
  - It contains the superficial fat compartments and the retinacular cutis extension of the "true" osseocutaneous retaining ligaments.
- **Layer 5** is the skin.

1.2 The Birthday Cake Analogy (The Layers of the Face)

A relatable analogy is comparing the facial layers to a two-tiered birthday cake. The platter of the cake is the facial skeleton, which undergoes resorption and alteration during the aging process. The first layer of cake is the "sub-SMAS" layer containing the deep facial fat compartments, potential spaces (i.e., upper temporal space aka interfascial plane, prezygomatic space, deep pyriform space), and the origins of the "true" osseocutaneous retaining ligaments (i.e., main zygomatic retaining ligament, orbital retaining ligament, zygomaticocutaneous retaining ligaments, mandibular osseocutaneous retaining ligament, platysma mandibular ligament). The middle layer of icing is the SMAS layer. In several locations in the face, the vasculature is commonly intertwined within the confines of SMAS layer and its analogues such as the superficial temporal fascia.

The top layer of cake is the "supra-SMAS" plane that contains the superficial fat compartments of the face, which are divided by vascular septae as well as the retinacular cutis of the facial retaining ligaments. One could consider the structure of the osseocutaneous retaining ligaments as a tree. In the deep layer of the face, the ligament is robust and compact like the trunk of a tree. As the ligament traverses superficial through the SMAS to eventually insert onto the skin the ligament "arborizes" into a branching pattern titled the retinacular cutis.

The top layer of icing is the skin which contains topographic anatomy reflecting the deeper layers of the face and their respective anatomical structures (i.e., lid–cheek junction, nasojugal groove, nasolabial fold, marionette crease) (▸ Fig. 1.5, ▸ Fig. 1.6, ▸ Fig. 1.7, ▸ Fig. 1.8).

1.3 The SMAS as a "Depth Gauge"

As the facial injector navigates the anatomy of the face, consideration should be given to the interplay and/or symphony of structures that contribute to each three-dimensional subunit in the face. For example, the injector can use the SMAS as a depth gauge to predictably access the deep layer of the face or as a stopping point to remain in the subcutaneous layer of the face. Then the injector can target specified fat compartments and/or potential spaces building between or within the facial retaining ligaments while exercising the appropriate amount of caution to avoid the vessels and lymphatics.

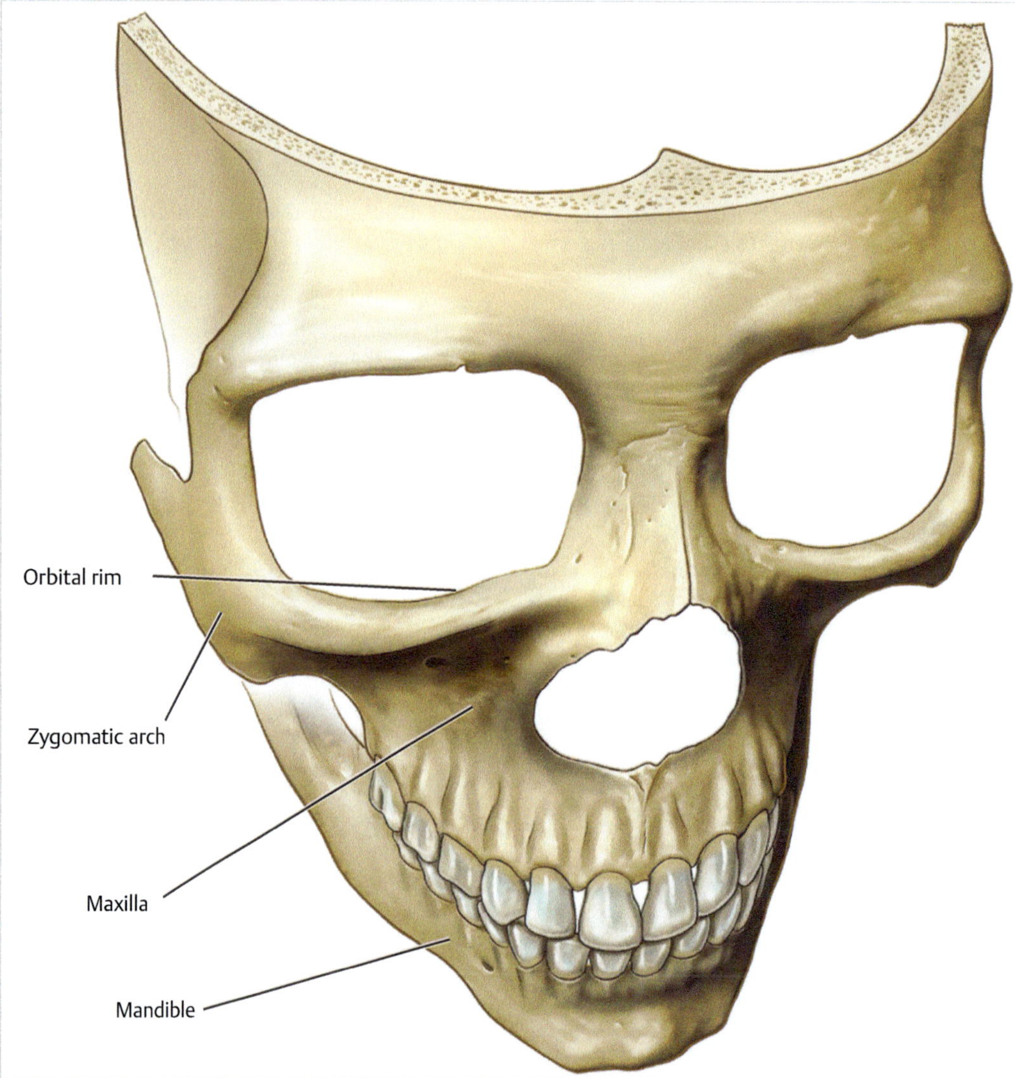

Fig. 1.1 Anatomic illustration of the facial skeleton. © Dr. Levent Efe, CMI.

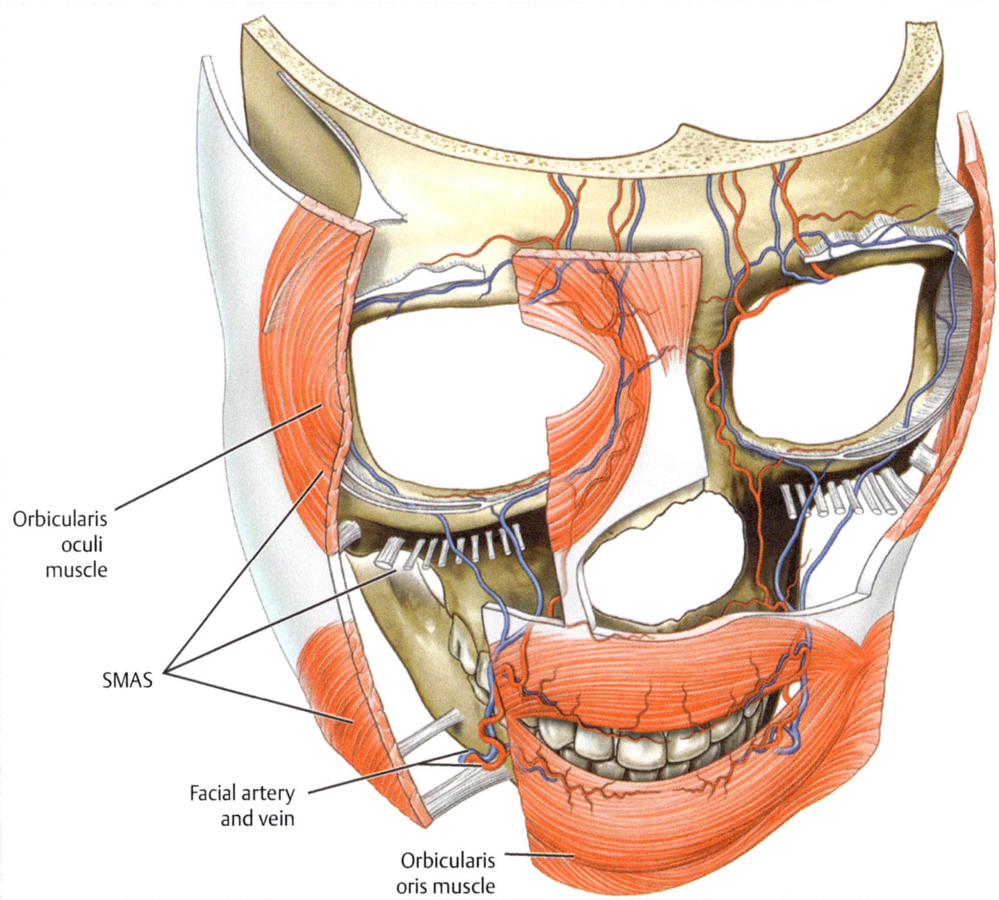

Fig. 1.2 Anatomic illustration of layer 4 of the face, also known as the "sub-SMAS plane" that contains the deep fat compartments of the face, the origin of the osseocutaneous retaining ligaments, and the gliding potential spaces of the face. SMAS, superficial musculoaponeurotic system. © Dr. Levent Efe, CMI.

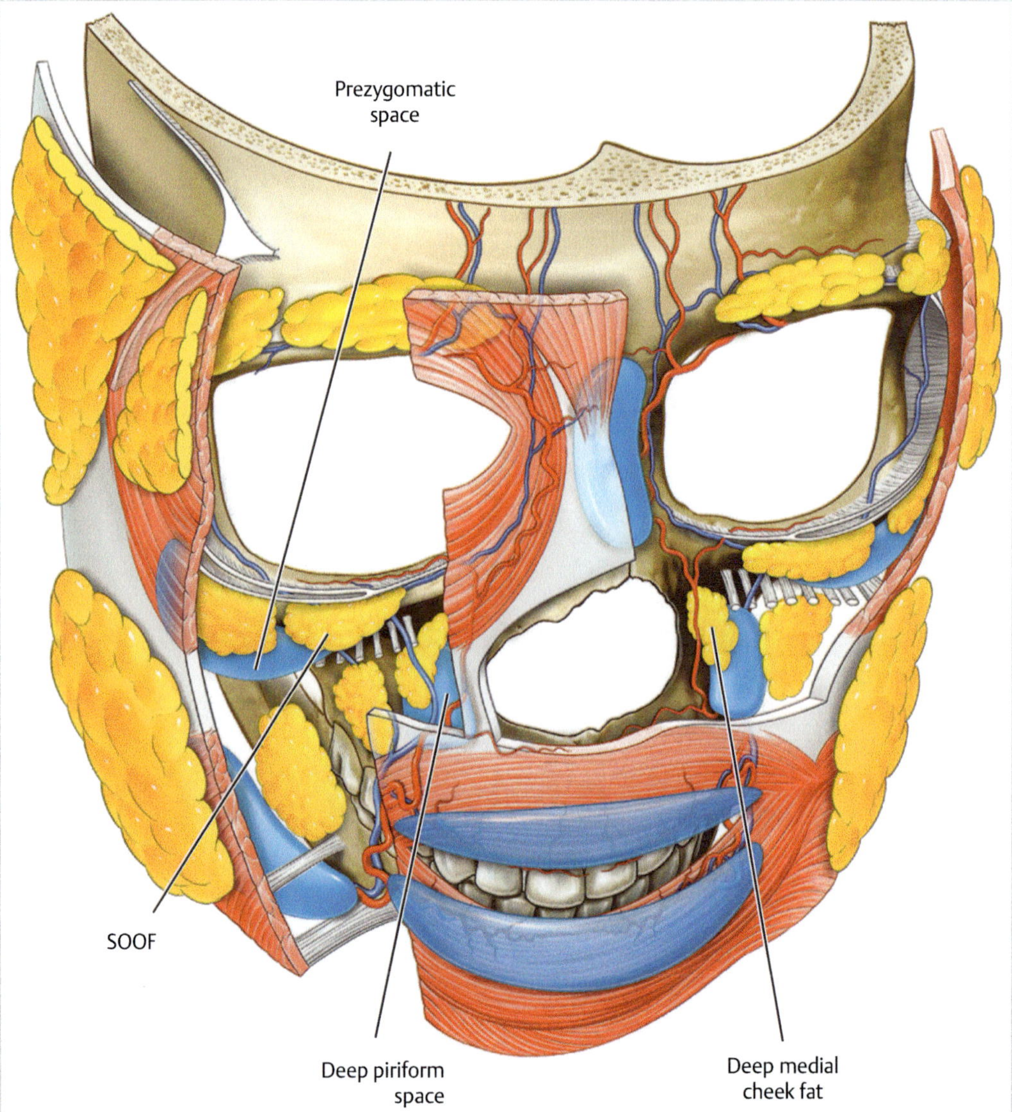

Fig. 1.3 Anatomic illustration of layer 3 of the face, also known as the "SMAS plane" that contains the muscles of facial animation as well as the arterial vasculature of the face in certain locations. SOOF, suborbicularis oculi fat. © Dr. Levent Efe, CMI.

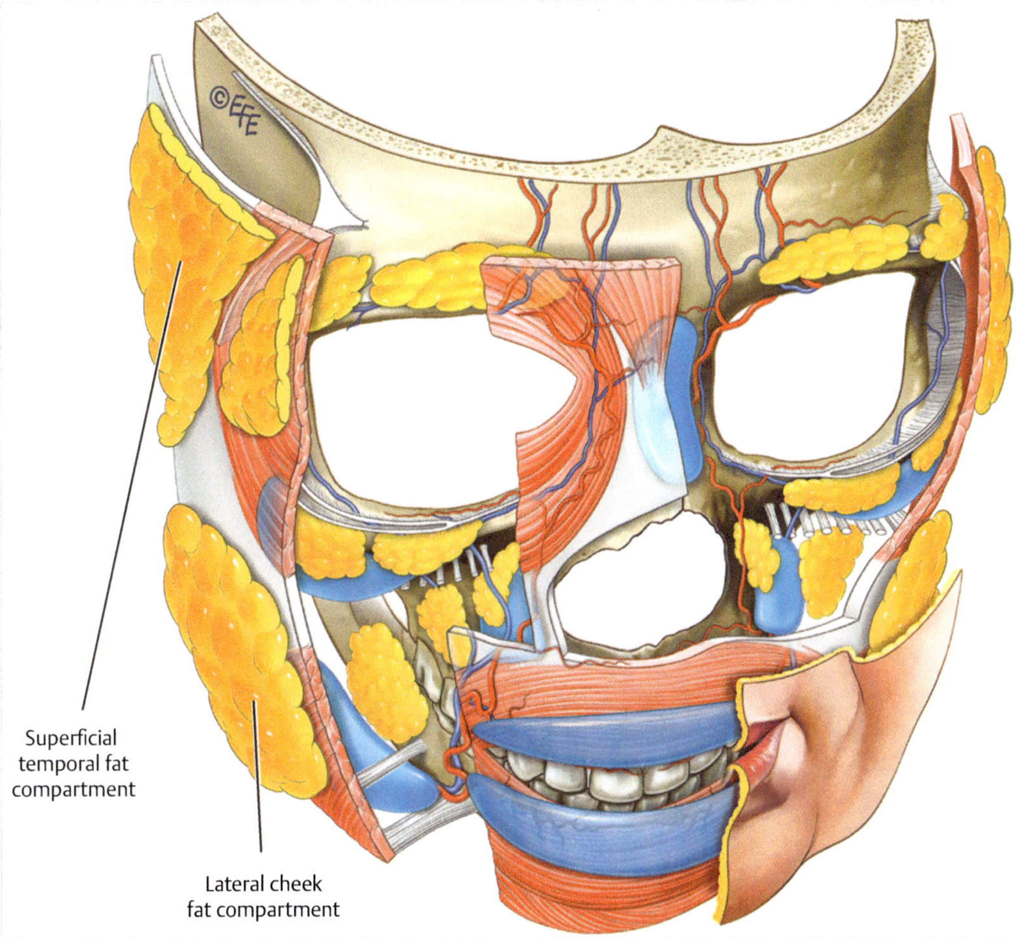

Fig. 1.4 Anatomic illustration of layer 2 of the face containing the superficial fat compartments and the branching retinacular cutis of the osseocutaneous retaining ligaments. © Dr. Levent Efe, CMI.

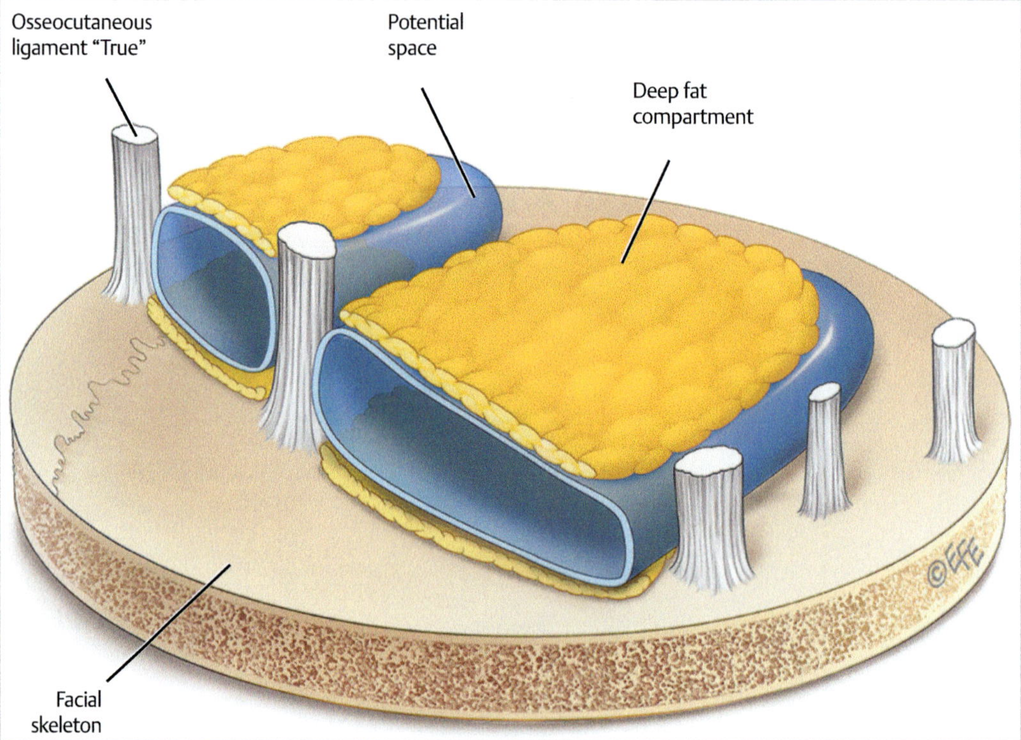

Fig. 1.5 Anatomic illustration with "cake layer" analogy demonstrating layer 4 of the face, also known as the "sub-SMAS plane" that contains the deep fat compartments of the face, the origin of the osseocutaneous retaining ligaments, and the gliding potential spaces of the face. © Dr. Levent Efe, CMI.

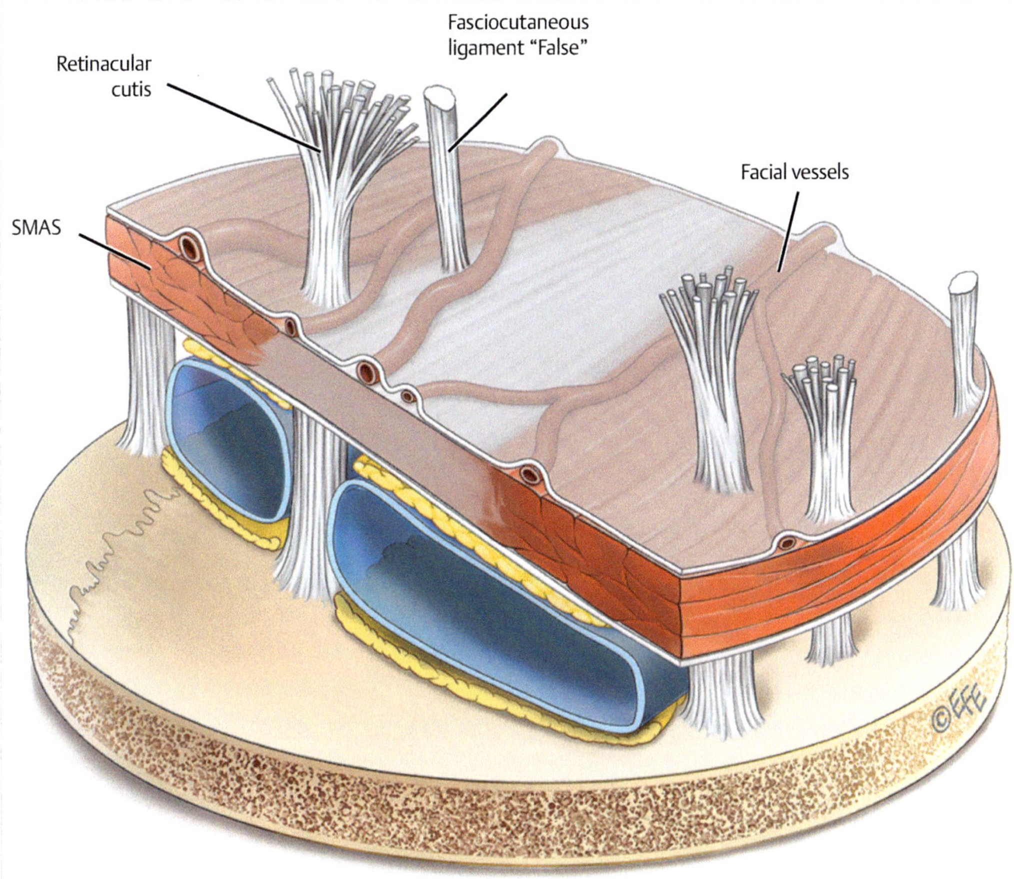

Fig. 1.6 Anatomic illustration with "cake layer" analogy demonstrating layer 3 of the face, also known as the "SMAS plane" that contains the muscles of facial animation as well as the arterial vasculature of the face in certain locations. SMAS, superficial musculoaponeurotic system. © Dr. Levent Efe, CMI.

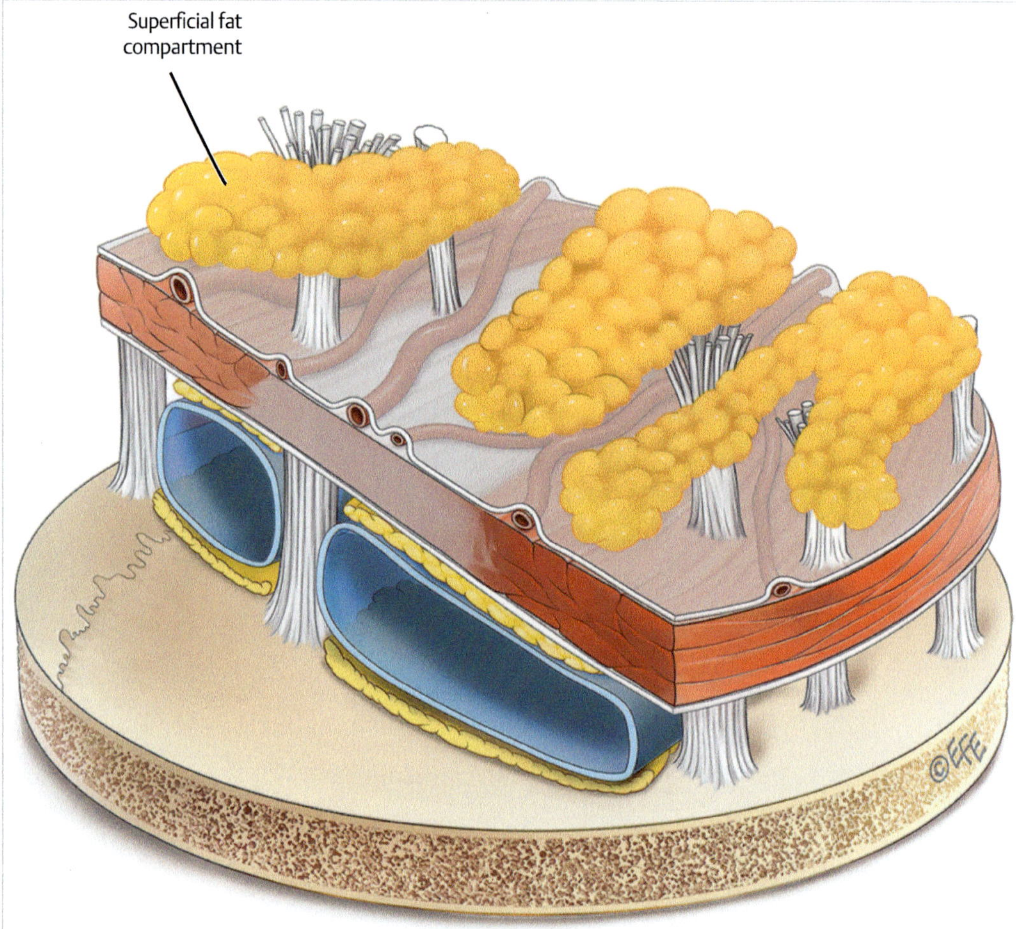

Fig. 1.7 Anatomic illustration with "cake layer" analogy demonstrating layer 2 of the face containing the superficial fat compartments and the branching retinacular cutis of the osseocutaneous retaining ligaments. © Dr. Levent Efe, CMI.

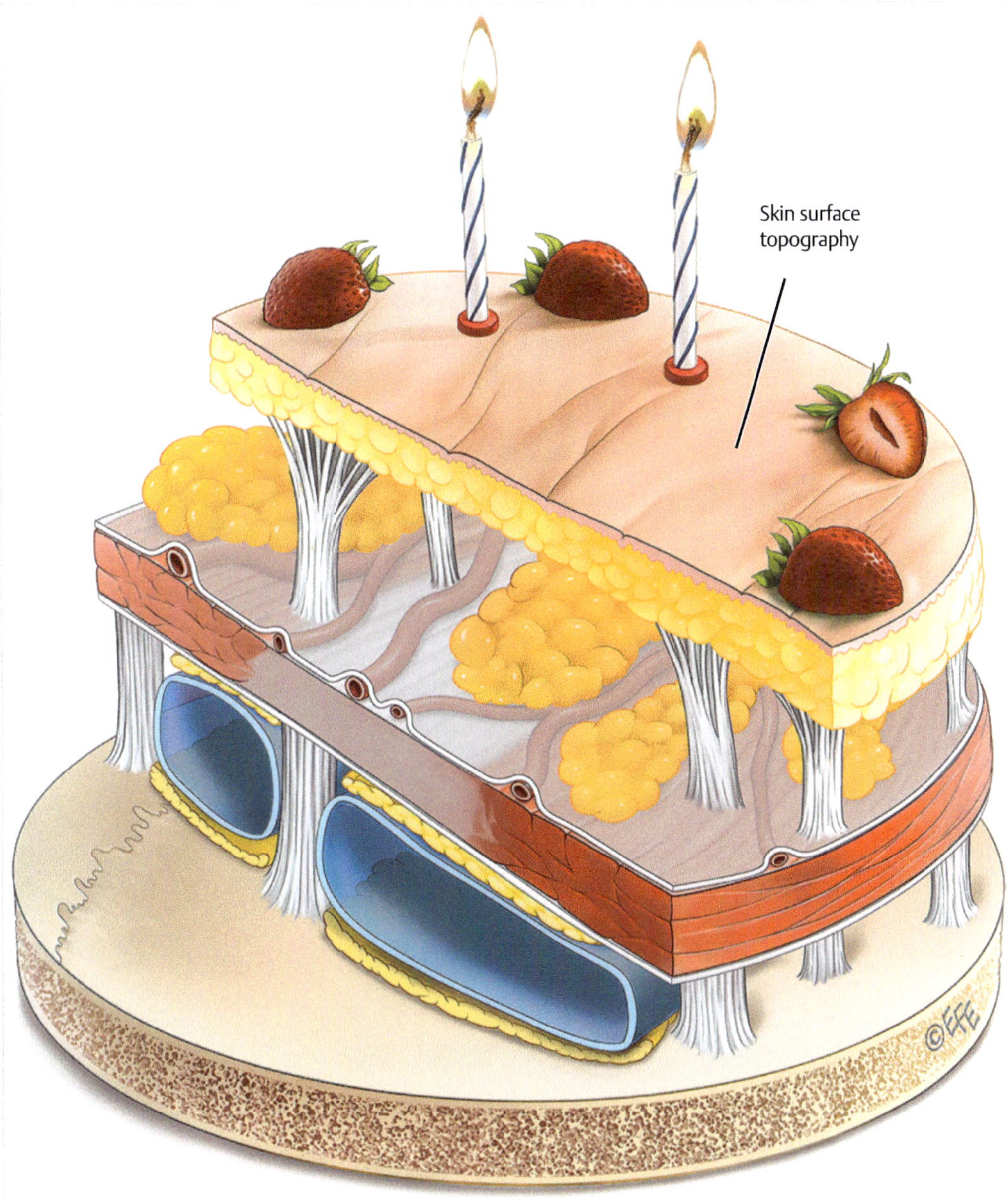

Fig. 1.8 Anatomic illustration with "cake layer" analogy demonstrating layer 1 of the face, which contains the skin and the associated surface topography that results from cutaneous insertions of the osseocutaneous retaining ligaments (i.e., lid–cheek junction and nasojugal groove) as well as other shadowing and contour changes that result from aging anatomy and facial shape alterations. © Dr. Levent Efe, CMI.

These anatomical concepts can be applied to the various aesthetic subunits of the face and aid the injector as to navigate desired targets and avoid potential danger zones during clinical injection.

Suggested Readings

Lamb J, Surek C. Facial Volumization: An Anatomic Approach. 1st ed. New York, NY: Thieme Medical Publishers; 2017

Mendelson B, Wong CH. Anatomy of the aging face. In: Neligan PC, ed. Plastic Surgery. Philadelphia, PA: Elsevier; 2013:78-92

Pessa J, Rohrich R. Facial Topography: Clinical Anatomy of the Face. St. Louis, MO: Quality Medical Publishing; 2012

Surek C. Facial Anatomy for Filler Injection: The Superficial Musculoaponeurotic System (SMAS) Is Not Just for Facelifting.Clin Plast Surg. 2019;46(4):603-612

Walker L, Cetto R. Facial Ageing and Injection Anatomy. 1st ed. UK Book Publishing; 2021

Chapter 2

Layered Anatomy of the Upper Face

2

2 Layered Anatomy of the Upper Face

Abstract
The upper face contains the temple, forehead, and glabella. With age, the temporal fossa is visualized due to soft tissue change and atrophy. Injection technique for temple volumization can be performed in multiple locations. Glabellar vasculature communicates closely with the ophthalmic vasculature. A comprehensive understating of upper facial vasculature is critical for the facial injector. This chapter will describe the three-dimensional layering of the temple, outlining possible targets for injection procedures as well as the vascular anatomy of the temple and glabellar regions. Anatomical descriptions are then complemented by detailed ultrasound visuals and technique pearls when imaging the upper face anatomy.

Keywords: Superficial temporal fascia, deep temporal fascia, superior temporal septum, inferior temporal septum, intermediate temporal fat pad, superficial temporal fat compartment, superficial temporal artery, supratrochlear artery, supraorbital artery, upper temporal space, interfascial plane

2.1 Temple

The layers of the temple are complex. A multilevel approach is often warranted when performing temple volumization procedures. The bony temple hollow becomes uncamouflaged with age. There is minimal bony change in the temporal fossa with age. Soft tissue atrophy of the temporalis muscle and intermediate temporal fat pad unveils the anterior–inferior bony trough of the temple fossa over time.

In this chapter, we will describe the temple layer by layer from deep to superficial. The temple fossa is composed of the parietal, temporal, frontal, and sphenoid bones. The first layer in the temple is the temporal extension of the buccal fat pad. Next is the temporalis muscle, which is covered the deep layer of deep temporal fascia (D-DTF). The deep and middle temporal arteries travel on the deep surface of the temporalis muscle and form a robust arterial network. The anterior deep temporal arteries are 1.5 to 2 cm lateral to the lateral orbital rim; therefore, deep supraperiosteal injections are recommended within 1 cm of the lateral orbital rim to avoid the deep temporal arteries which have connections to the ophthalmic vasculature. The D-DTF is a continuation of the periosteum of the frontal bone (▶ Fig. 2.1, ▶ Fig. 2.2).

The deep temporal fascia (DTF) splits into a deep layer (D-DTF) and superficial layer (S-DTF) which wraps around the intermediate temporal fat pad. This has been described as a potential target for volumization. However, the fat pad often contains a branch of the middle temporal vein. It is recommended to access this fat pad through direct visual guidance only with ultrasound to ensure accuracy and avoid vascular sequalae. The middle temporal vein runs 20 mm superior to the zygomatic arch and joins the superficial temporal vein above the level of the arch (▶ Fig. 2.3, ▶ Fig. 2.4).

> **Key Point**
>
> The muscles of mastication (masseter and temporalis) have a different embryologic origin than the muscles of facial expression. Therefore, the masseter and temporalis are covered by deep facial fascia whereas the muscles of facial expression (mimetic muscles) are commonly invested in the superficial facial fascia also known as the superficial musculoaponeurotic system (SMAS).

The next layer is an open gliding potential space called the upper temporal space, also known as the interfascial plane. This potential space is bounded superiorly and inferiorly by fascial septa. These septa travel from the DTF to superficial temporal fascia (STF), which is continuation of the SMAS in the temple. The superior boundary is the superior temporal septum (STS). This STS runs along the bony temporal crest, which can be easily palpated during clinical assessment. The inferior boundary is the inferior temporal septum (ITS). Clinically, this can be marked on the surface of the skin using an oblique line from the superior lateral orbital rim to the root of the helix. The ITS is an important landmark as it often stabilizes rami branches of the frontal branch of the facial nerve as well as anterior arterial branches of the superficial temporal artery (STA) (▶ Fig. 2.5, ▶ Fig. 2.6).

The next layer after the upper temporal space (aka interfascial plane) is the STF, which is synonymous with the SMAS. It has been shown that the arterial branches of the STA often travel within the

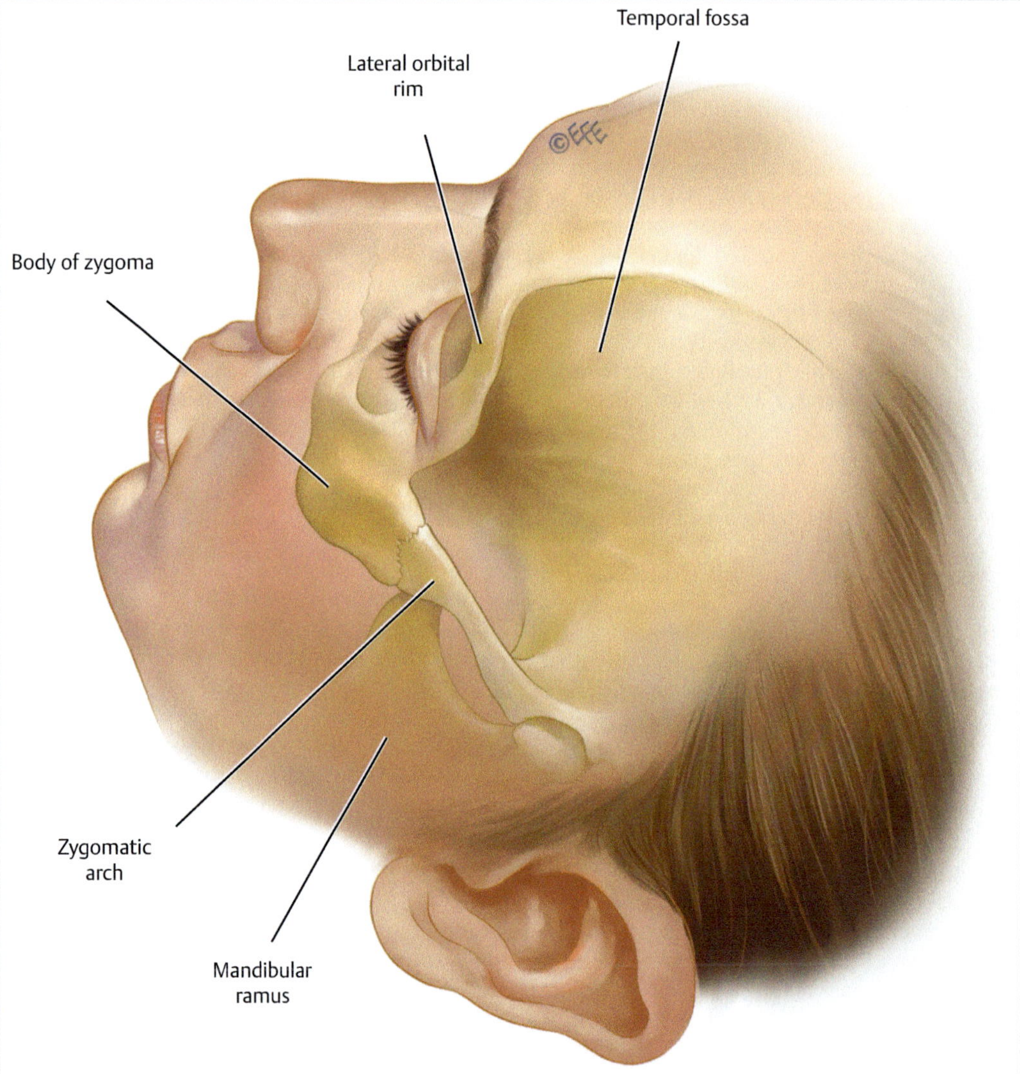

Fig. 2.1 Anatomic illustration of the temporal fossa. This fossa is camouflaged by soft tissue fullness in the youthful face but becomes more noticeable with age as soft tissue changes and atrophy occur. © Dr. Levent Efe, CMI.

confines of the SMAS. This is an important clinical pearl of the injector when determining volumization targets in the temple. When the STA reaches the temporal crest, it courses superficially and commonly anastomoses with supraorbital arterial branches creating a vascular connection between the temple and ophthalmic vasculature. Superficial to the SMAS lies the superficial temporal fat compartment. This compartment is prone to atrophy with aging. This compartment can serve as good target for volumization procedures often resulting in a direct 1:1 change in surface topography following injection (▸ Fig. 2.7, ▸ Fig. 2.8).

Key Point

The anterior branch of the STA often travels in close proximity to the ITS; therefore, caution must be taken when injecting near this region. Additionally, the STA and its branches often travel within the SMAS. Therefore, it is recommended to stay superficial or deep to the SMAS during injections to avoid interaction with the vasculature within the SMAS.

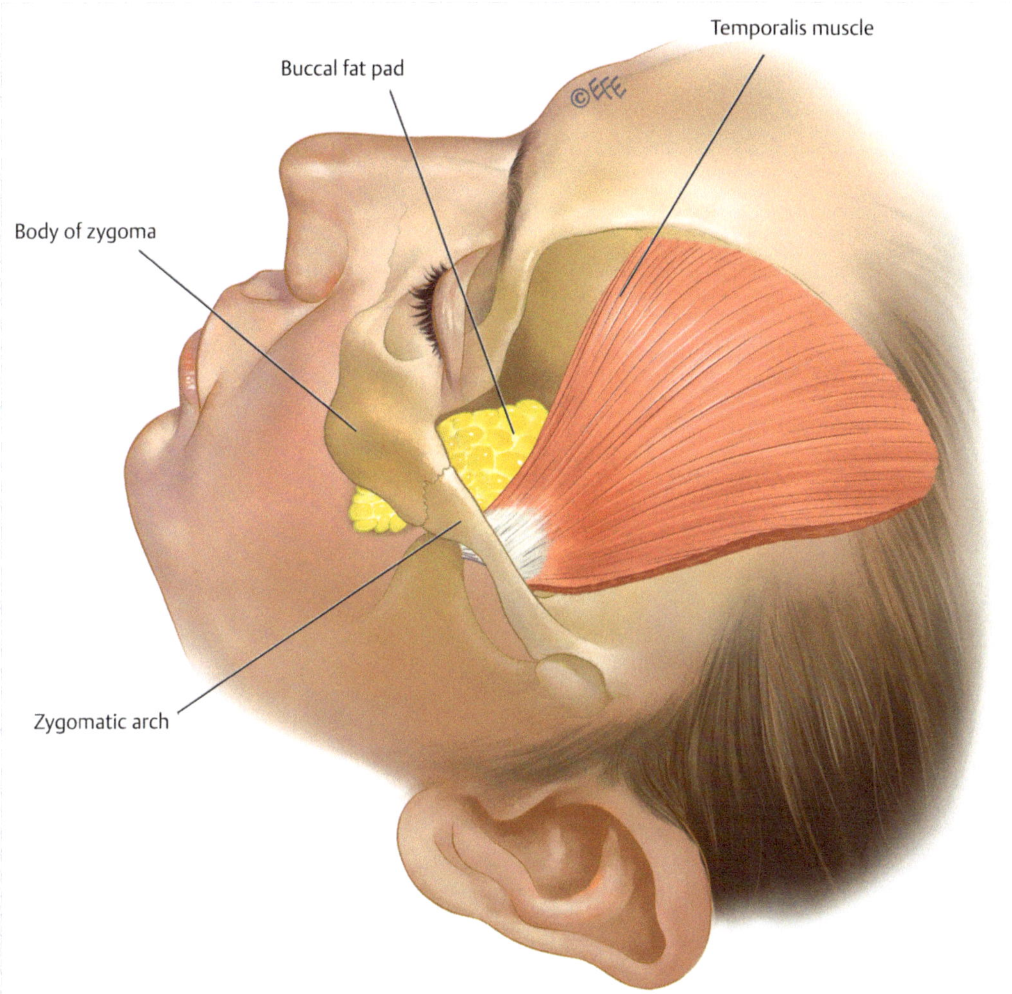

Fig. 2.2 Anatomic illustration of the temporalis muscle (i.e., muscle of mastication) and the temporal extension of the buccal fat pad. © Dr. Levent Efe, CMI.

The final layer in the temple is the skin. Be mindful that atrophy of the soft tissues and thinning of the skin can make superficial injections challenging; therefore, attention should given to ensure the injector stays above or below and not within the SMAS during clinical injection.

2.2 Glabella

The glabella is comprised of multiple brow depressor muscles including the procerus muscle, corrugator muscles, depressor supercilii muscles, and orbicularis oculi muscles. The supratrochlear neurovascular bundle is located approximately 1.7 to 2.2 cm from the midline passing through or superficial to the corrugator muscle. The artery travels within the glabellar crease in 50% of cases or within 3 mm lateral to the crease in the other 50%. The bundle travels superiorly on the periosteum in the lower third of the forehead (1.5–2.5 cm above the superior orbital rim), then ascends into the frontalis muscle in the middle third of the forehead, and eventually courses subcutaneously in the upper third of the forehead.

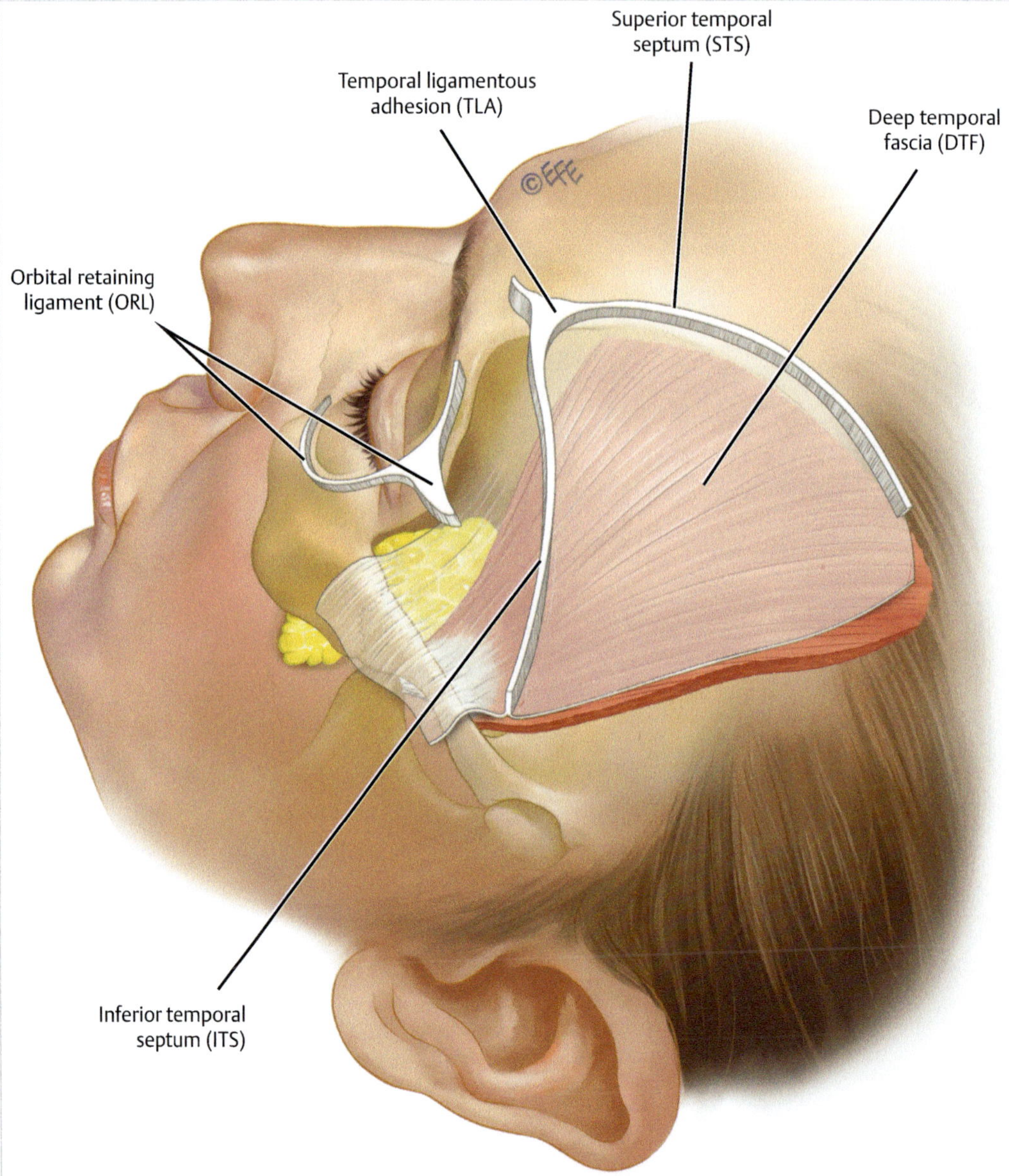

Fig. 2.3 Anatomic illustration of the deep temporal fascia covering the temporalis muscle, which is a continuation of the periosteum of the frontal bone. The superior and inferior temporal septa traverse from deep temporal fascia to superficial temporal fascia and coalesce at the temporal ligamentous adhesion (TLA) located at the superior lateral orbital rim. © Dr. Levent Efe, CMI.

The supraorbital neurovascular bundle is located approximately 2.5 cm from the midline and follows a similar depth pathway as the supratrochlear neurovascular bundle. Subcutaneously in the midline in 65% of cases, the central artery arises from the dorsal nasal artery and the paracentral artery arises from the angular artery forming an anastomotic network in the glabellar region. Overall, glabellar vasculature has several direct connections to the ophthalmic vasculature. The glabella is the second most common location of filler injection vision compromise (▶ Fig. 2.9).

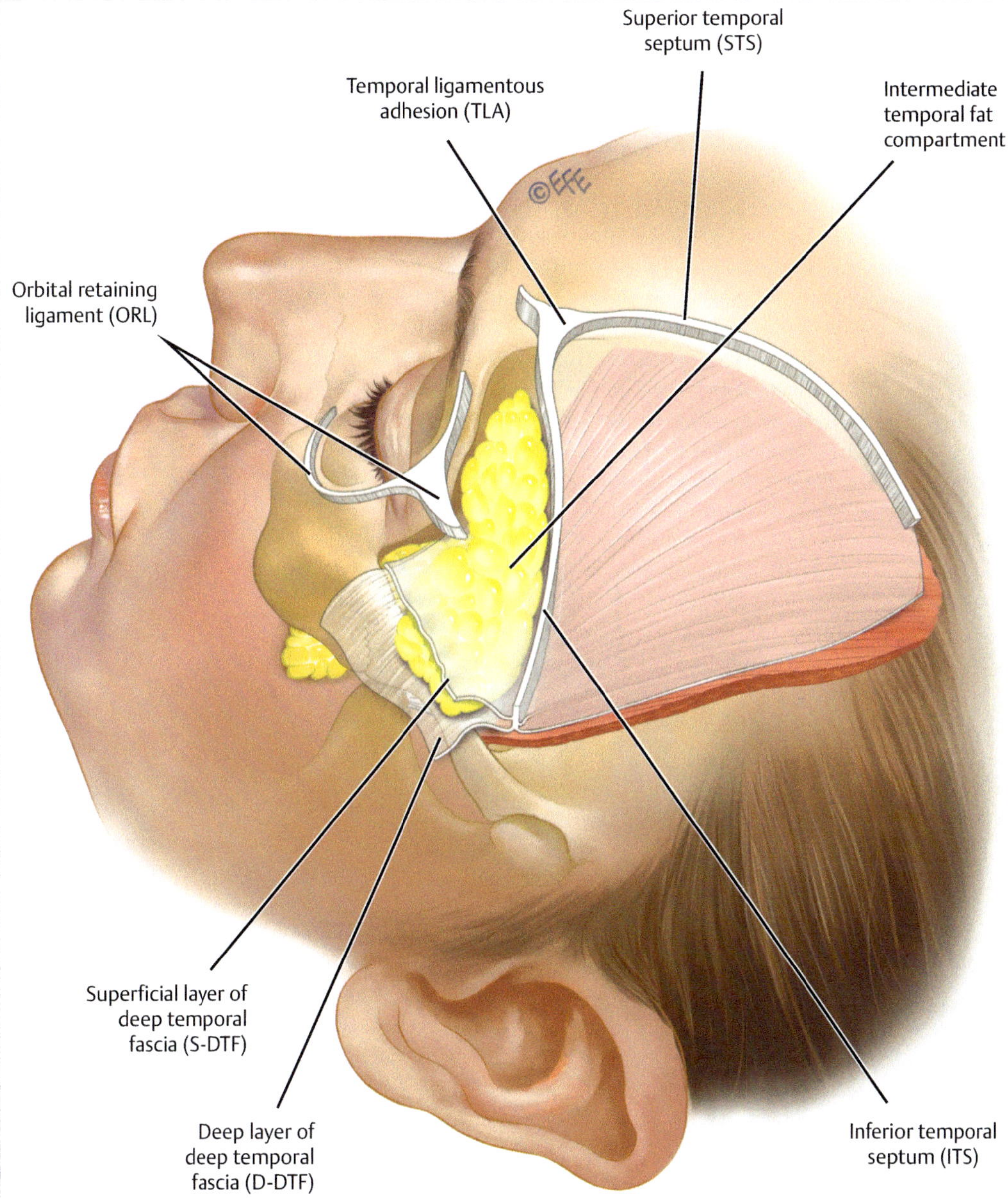

Fig. 2.4 Anatomic illustration of the intermediate temporal fat pad, which is located over the anterior–inferior trough of the temporal fossa and is wrapped by the superficial layer of deep temporal fascia (S-DTF) and deep layer of deep temporal fascia (D-DTF). © Dr. Levent Efe, CMI.

2.3 Ultrasound Anatomy and Technique for the Temple

Imaging of the temple region is essential to accurately place filler in the correct injection plane and to evaluate filler and complications. An 18- or 20-MHz probe is suitable for imaging all the anatomy with the exception of the deep temporal arteries. Although some deep temporal arteries can be visualized with the higher frequency

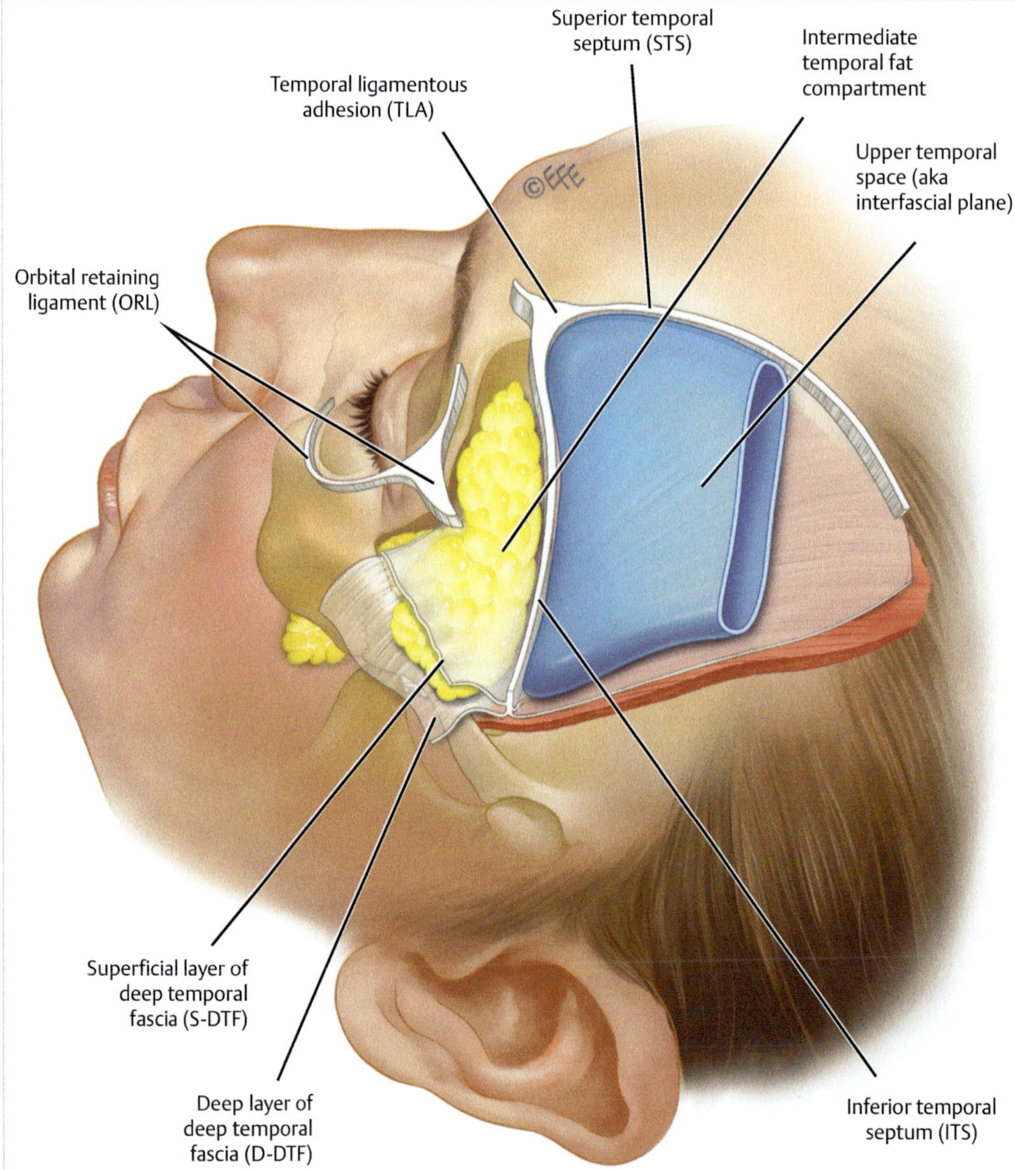

Fig. 2.5 Anatomic illustration of the upper temporal space (aka interfascial plane), which is located between the deep temporal fascia and the superficial temporal fascia (STF). © Dr. Levent Efe, CMI.

probes, the 12-MHz probe is more consistently able to do so.

There are three positions of the probe that are routinely effective in the temple. A vertical probe can visualize a cross section of the anterior branch of the STA and all the layers of the temple. A horizontal probe is useful for evaluating the course of the anterior branch of the STA and the various layers of the temple, including a cross section of the deep temporal arteries. The higher the probe, the less likely it is to see the intermediate temporal fat pad. One other favorite position by the author (S.W.) is a slightly tilted vertical position of the probe, which lies parallel to the superior–lateral orbital rim. This enables a view of the course of the deep temporal arteries (▶ Fig. 2.10).

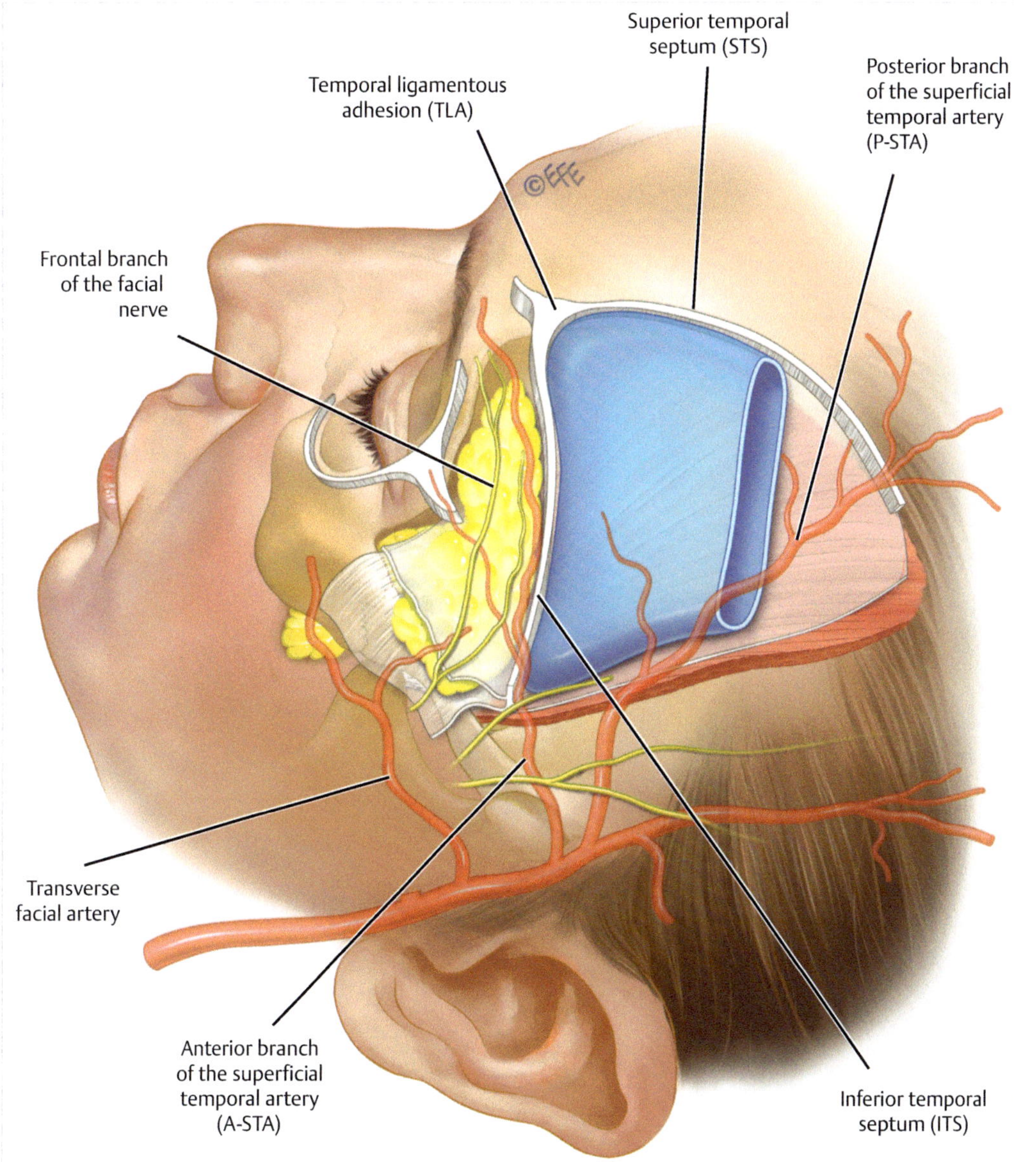

Fig. 2.6 Anatomic illustration of the superficial temporal artery (STA) and the frontal branch of the facial nerve. Note the anterior branch of the STA and a frontal branch facial nerve rami are running in proximity with the inferior temporal septum. An important relationship to note in the temple region. © Dr. Levent Efe, CMI.

Mapping of the temple should not be a prolonged process. For deep supraperiosteal injections, a mark should be placed at the intended injection site. Ultrasound of this area should be performed to evaluate whether the deep temporal artery is found on the periosteum directly beneath this point. If none is found, an injection is considered "safe" and the standard protocol of injection onto periosteum should be performed. This is considered "safe" mapping.

To map the anterior branch of the STA, a probe should be placed on or near the ITS. The artery is found to be within or in close proximity to this septum in > 80% of the time. This septum lies

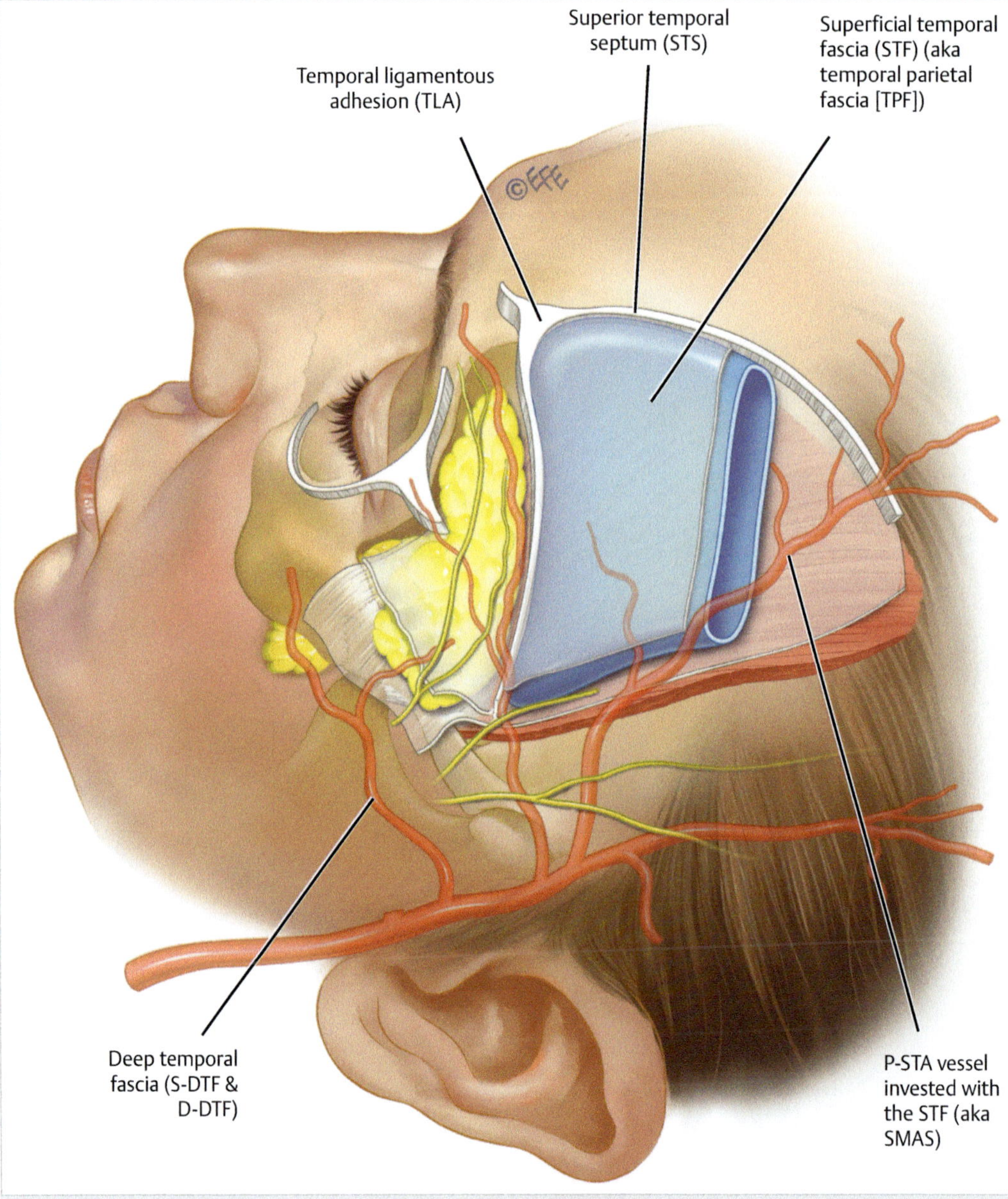

Fig. 2.7 Anatomic illustration of the superficial temporal fascia, which is synonymous with the superficial musculoaponeurotic system (SMAS). The superficial temporal artery branches commonly run within the superficial temporal fascia (STF). © Dr. Levent Efe, CMI.

between the superior orbital rim and the root of the helix. The artery will be found in the SMAS layer but can be extremely tortuous, leading to some portions but not the entirety of the vessel being visualized in some patients. In 37% of patients, the posterior STA is dominant making the anterior branch "insignificant."

Interfascial plane injection technique is effective for volumizing the temple. Confirming the plane using ultrasound should be a consideration for

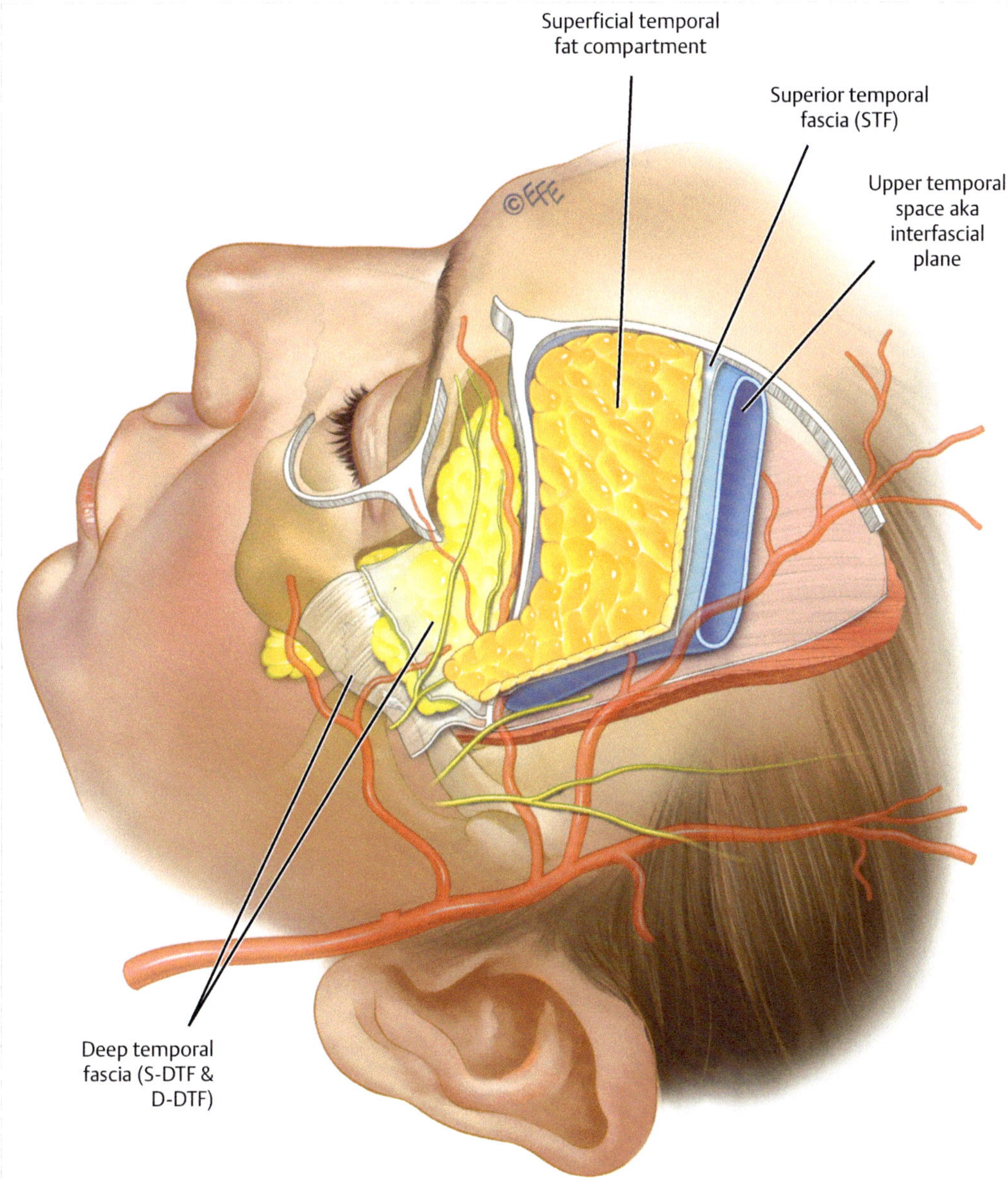

Fig. 2.8 Anatomic illustration of the superficial temporal fat compartment located superficial to the superficial temporal fascia (STF) and directly beneath the dermis of the temple skin. © Dr. Levent Efe, CMI.

additional patient safety. If the cannula position is difficult to ascertain with ultrasound, a small injection (0.3 cc) of saline can be performed to confirm location and expand the interfascial plane.

In this ultrasound view of the temple, the 18-MHz probe is placed vertically.

There are ten visible layers (▶ Fig. 2.11, ▶ Fig. 2.12, ▶ Fig. 2.13, ▶ Fig. 2.14, ▶ Fig. 2.15, ▶ Fig. 2.16, ▶ Fig. 2.17, ▶ Fig. 2.18, ▶ Fig. 2.19, ▶ Fig. 2.20):

1. Skin (epidermis + dermis)—gray.
2. Superficial fat pad (lateral temporal fat)—gold.

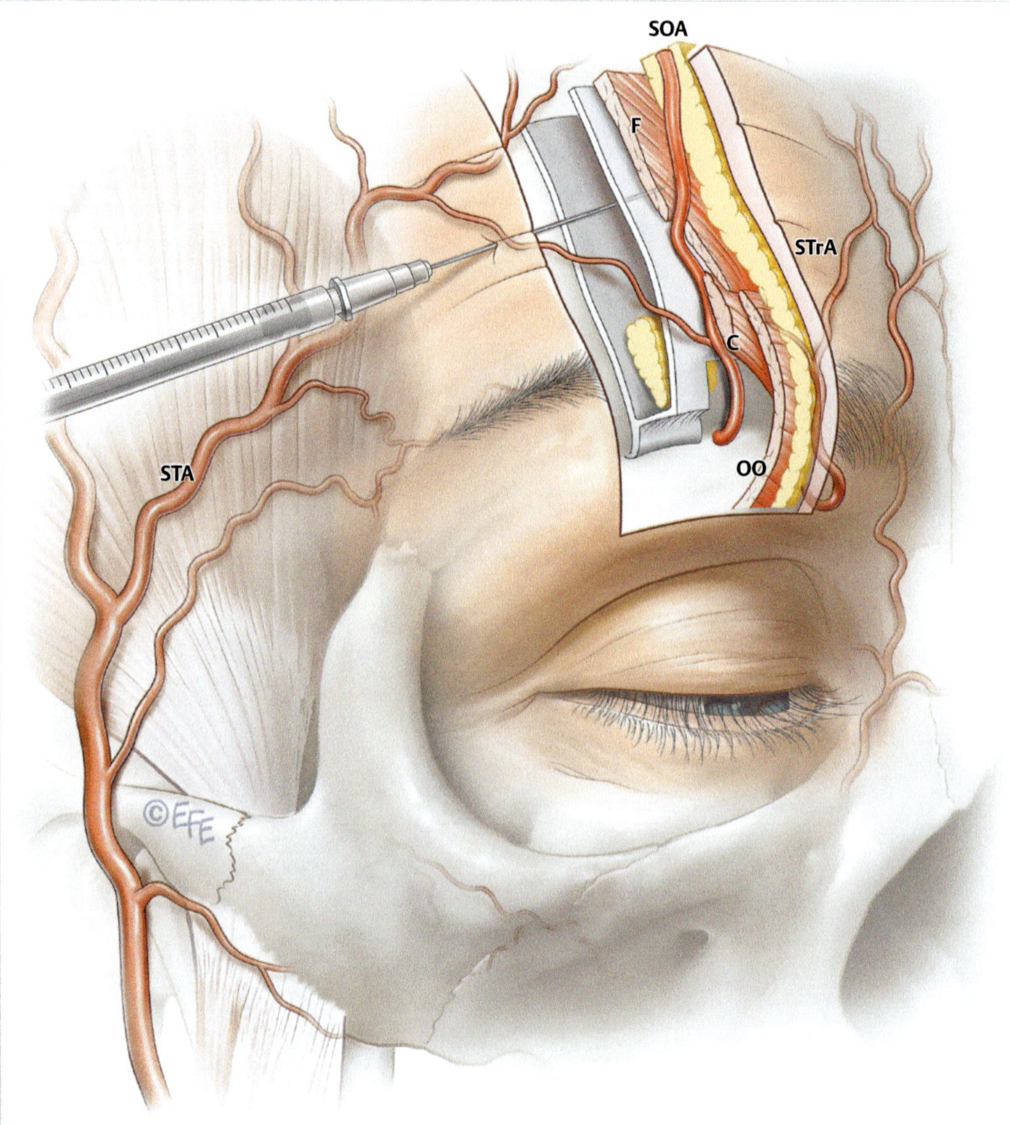

Fig. 2.9 Anatomical illustration of the connection between the superficial temporal artery (STA) and the supraorbital artery (SOA) and supratrochlear artery (STrA) which communicate with ophthalmic vasculature. When attempting forehead soft tissue filler injection, a preferred plane is subgaleal below the frontalis (F), corrugator (C), and orbicularis oculi (OO) muscles and in the middle or upper one-third of the forehead to avoid the SOA and STrA vessels that lie on the periosteum on the frontal bone. © Dr. Levent Efe, CMI.

3. SMAS/STF/Temporoparietal fascia—blue.
4. STA (anterior and posterior branches within the SMAS)—red.
5. Interfascial plane/Innominate fascia—yellow.
6. DTF—light blue.
7. S-DTF—violet.
8. Intermediate temporal fat pad—green.
9. D-DTF—brown.
10. Temporalis muscle—purple.
11. Temporal bone—pink.

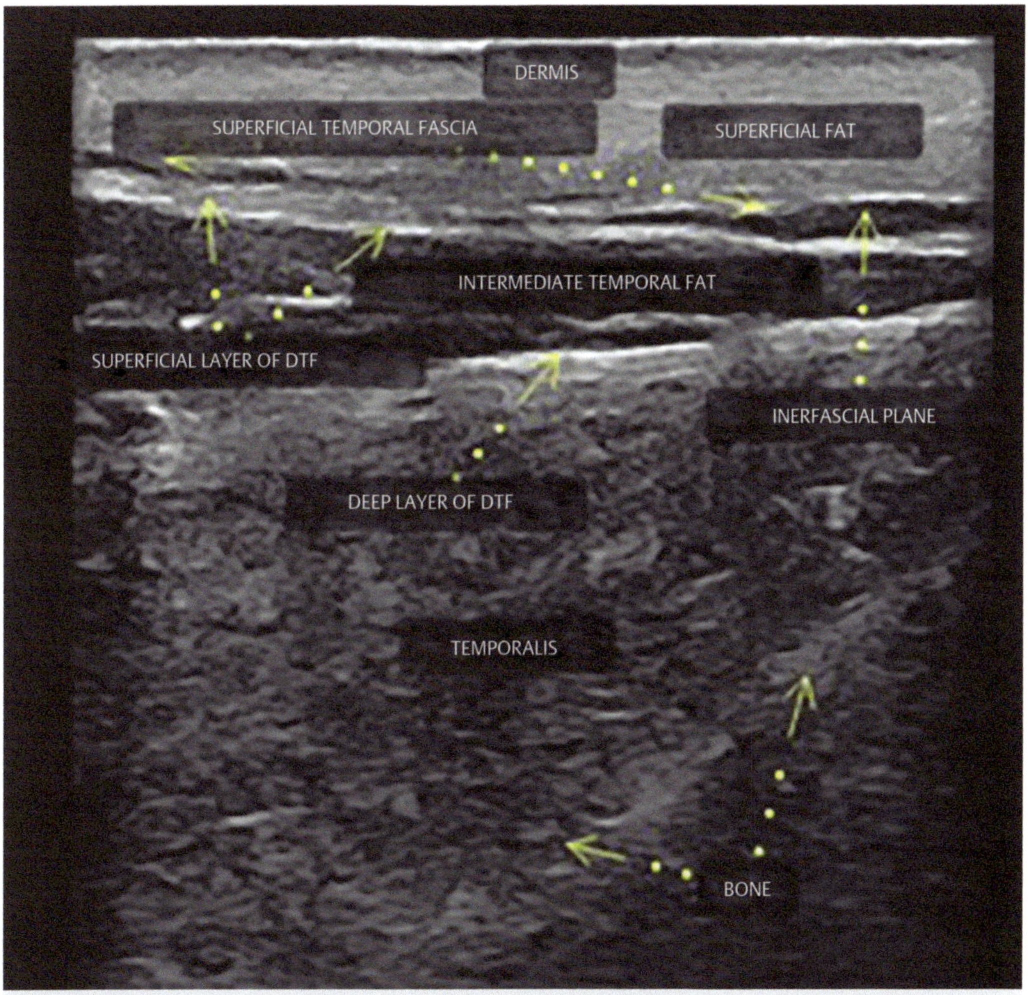

Fig. 2.10 Image obtained using a 20 MHz handheld probe. Note the two layers of the deep temporal fascia envelope the intermediate temporal fat pad. Also note the interfascial plane between the superficial temporal fascia and the superficial layer of the deep temporal fascia. (DTF = Deep temporal fascia).

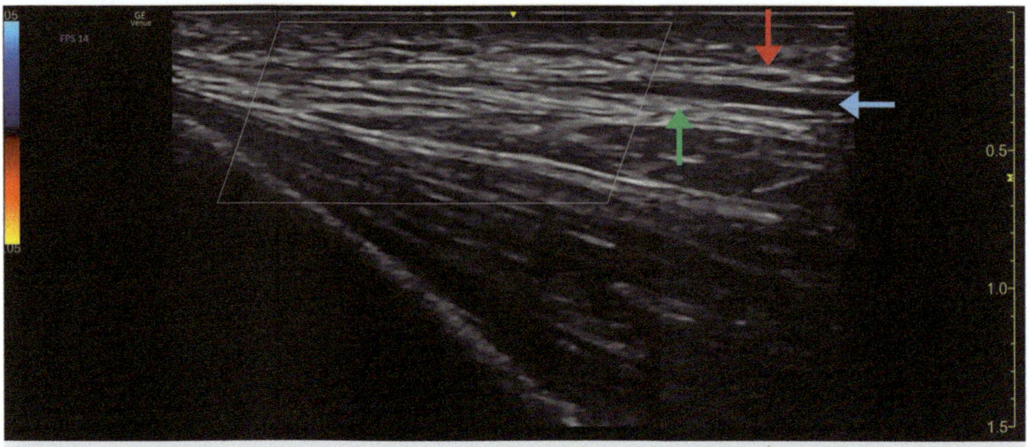

Fig. 2.11 Image obtained using a vertical 18-MHz probe. The interfascial plane is a potential space and is not always well visualized on ultrasound prior to filler placement. However, in the image, this space is easily seen (blue arrow). Superficial musculoaponeurotic system (SMAS) is shown with red arrow; superficial layer of deep temporal fascia is shown with green arrow.

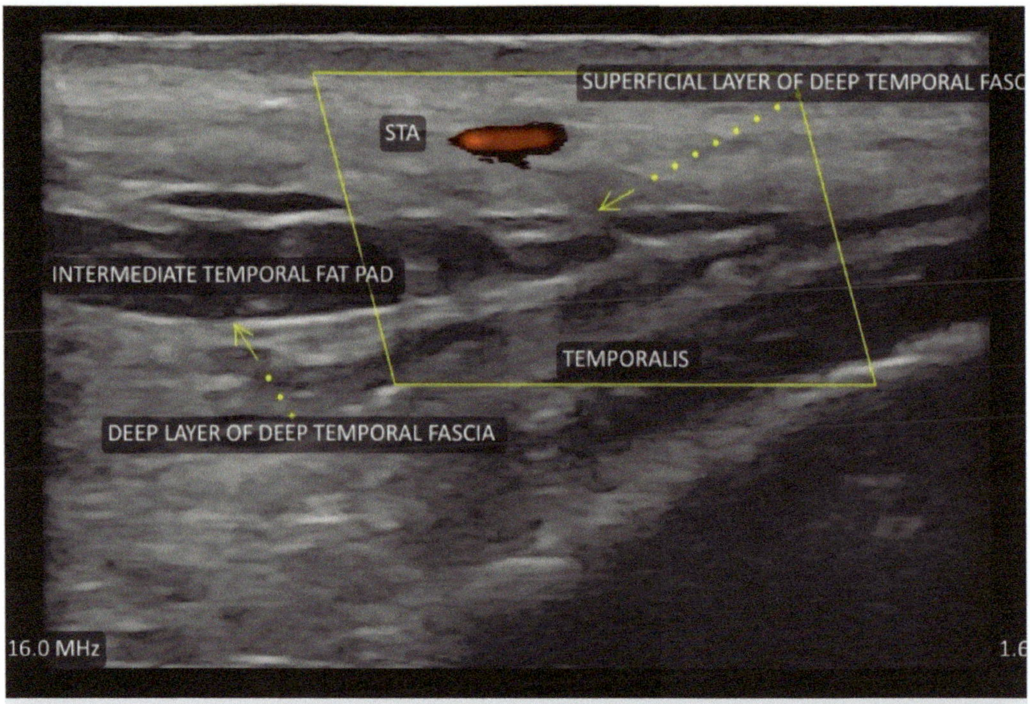

Fig. 2.12 Color duplex image using a vertical 20-MHz handheld probe. All the layers previously noted can be seen on this image. Note the differences in echogenicity of the superficial fat (superficial temporal fat pad) and the intermediate temporal fat pad, which can be attributed to differences in the fibrous content (collagen). The superficial musculoaponeurotic system (SMAS) layer (containing the superficial temporal artery [STA]) is less robust than the deep temporal fascia and therefore is less easily seen as a defined layer in some patients.

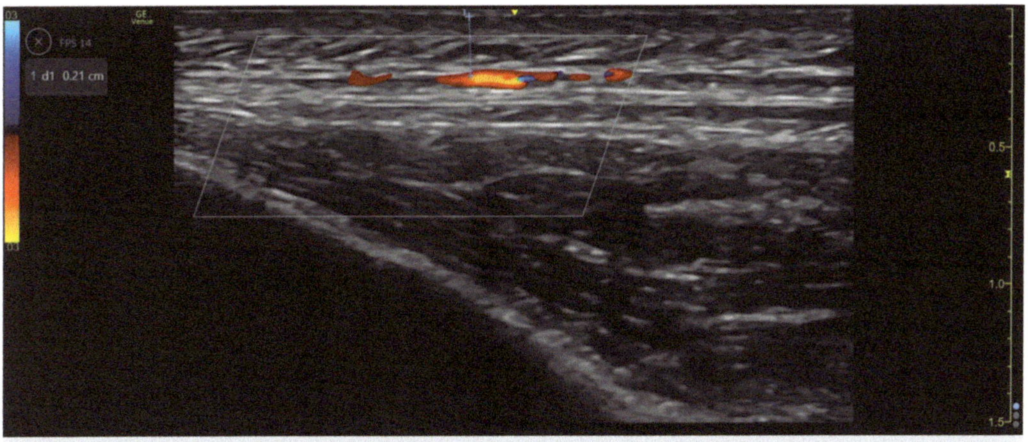

Fig. 2.13 Color Doppler image using a horizontal 18-MHz probe showing the anterior branch of the superficial temporal artery. It lies within the superficial musculoaponeurotic system (SMAS) layer and is often very tortuous making visualization of its full length difficult in most cases. It is a high-flow artery so velocity scale might need to be adjusted higher to avoid color aliasing, and color gain will often be set relatively low. In 37% of patients, the posterior branch is dominant, and the anterior branch is negligible. In > 80% of patients, the anterior branch of the superficial temporal artery will travel in the inferior temporal septum, which runs from the superior orbital rim to the root of the helix.

2.4 Injection Planes in the Temple

There are three planes routinely used for temporal injections.

2.4.1 First Injection Plane

The superficial temporal fat pad lies above the SMAS (i.e., superficial temporal fat compartment) and gives the most displacement of tissue per volume injected. The safest method of injection is using a cannula. Visible and palpable filler can be drawback for this layer of injection. Reconstitution of filler may decrease palpability and visibility of product injected in this tissue plane.

2.4.2 Second Injection Plane

The interfascial plane is another reliable option because it gives a fairly robust volumization with less risk of visible filler than the superficial injection layer. It lies below the SMAS/STA; however, the sentinel vein lies in this layer. Disruption of the vein can result in a hematoma if not recognized quickly, and extremely rarely, a pulmonary embolus is possible. This injection is safest if performed with cannulas.

2.4.3 Third Injection Plane

The deep injection on bone, "One up, One over" or "Gunshot" technique, is the most popular deep injection for the temples. It must be performed with a needle because of the need to pierce the thick DTF (which is a continuation of periosteum of the frontal bone). Its drawbacks are the dangers of intraarterial injection of the deep temporal artery (blindness or occlusion are possible), movement of filler throughout the temporalis over time due to chewing and talking, and the need for larger volume of filler to achieve similar clinical results as the other injection planes relative to surface topography changes.

In a paper by Casabona et al, the above three techniques were compared.

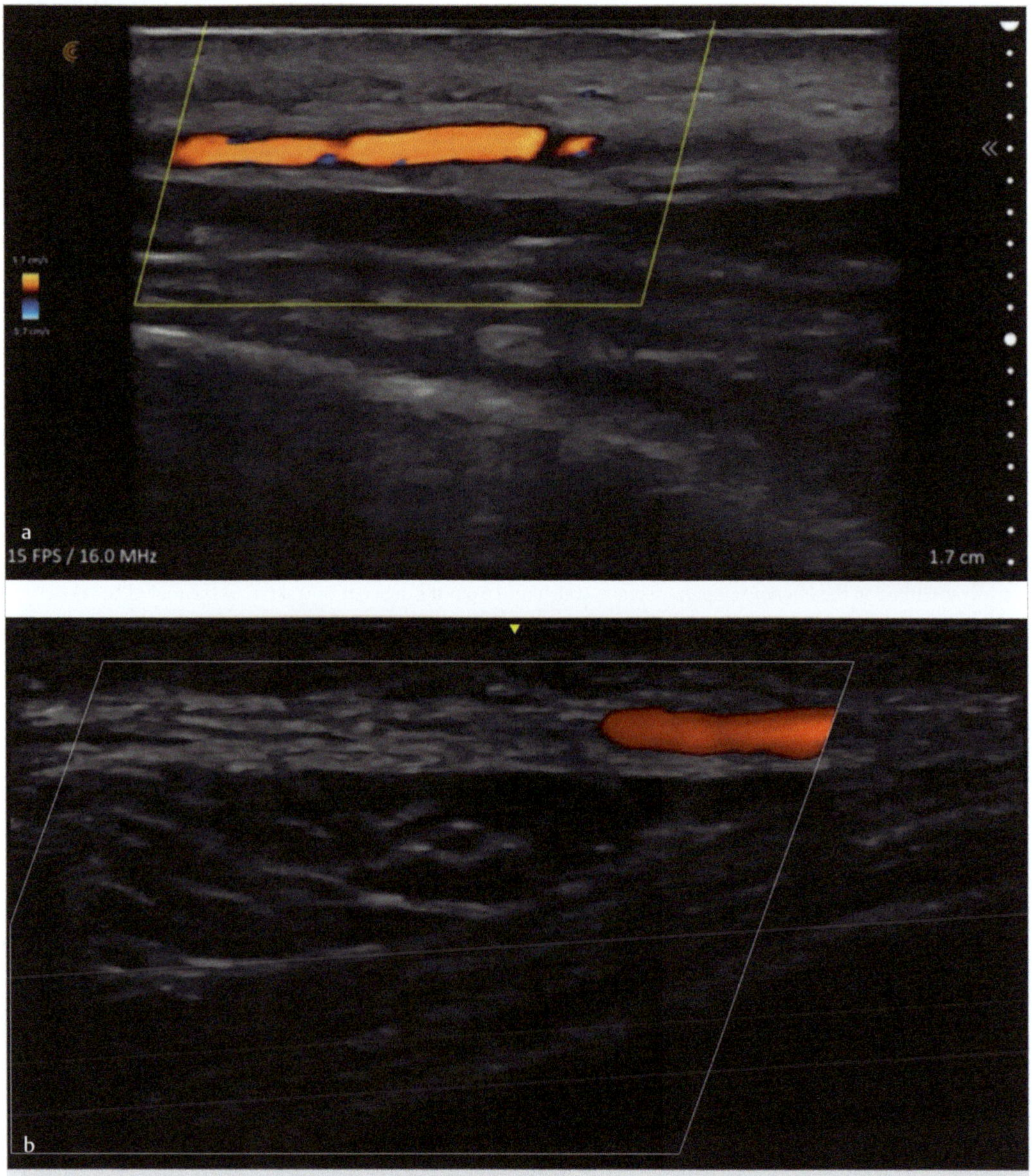

Fig. 2.14 (a) Color duplex image using a 20-MHz handheld probe in horizontal position. Note the position of the anterior branch of the superficial temporal artery just below the superficial temporal fat compartment in the superficial musculoaponeurotic system (SMAS) layer (aka superficial temporal fascia). **(b)** 12 MHz probe in horizontal position showing the superficial temporal artery in the SMAS or superficial temporal fascia layer.

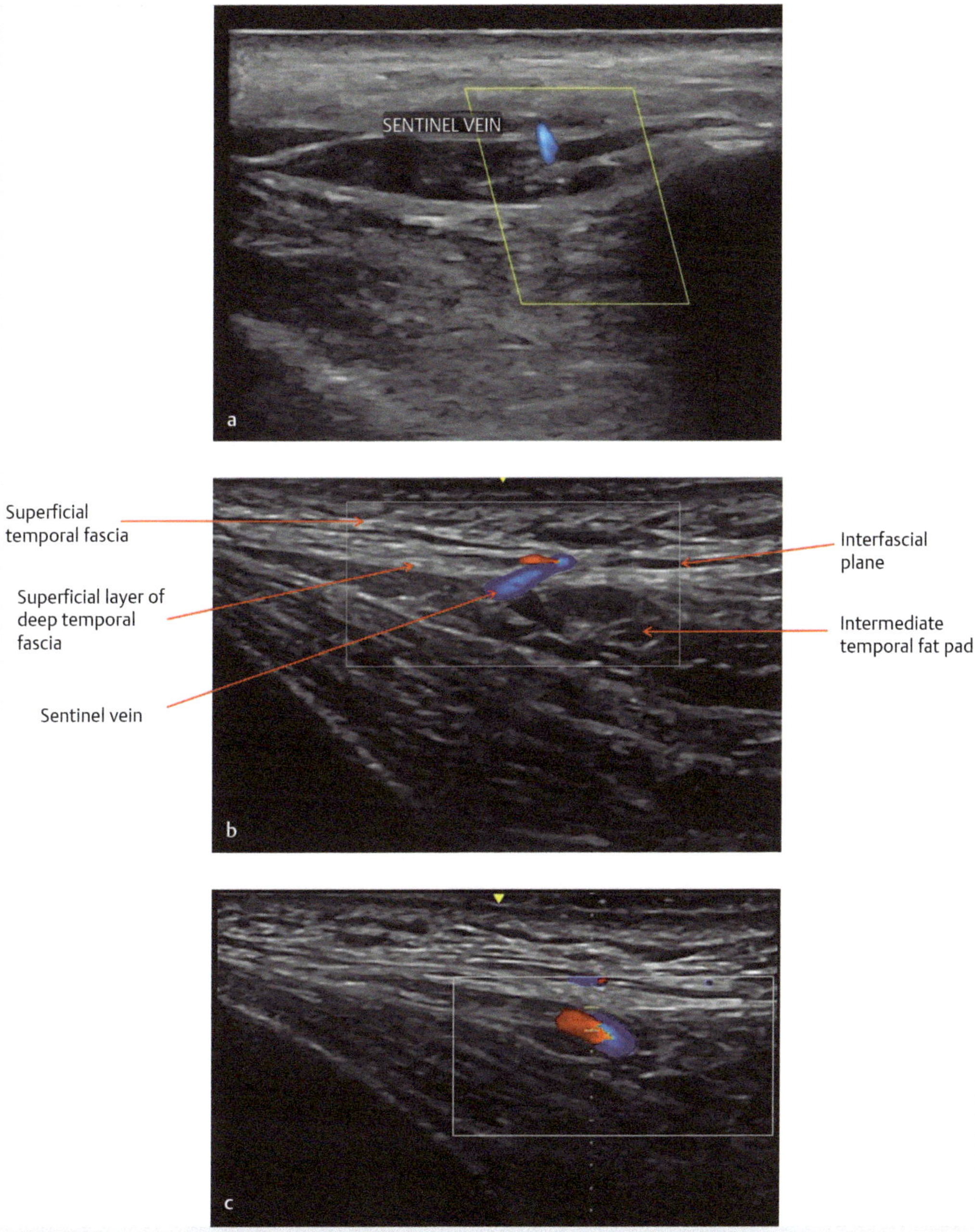

Fig. 2.15 **(a)** Image obtained using a vertical 20-MHz handheld probe showing the sentinel vein. This vein collects all the superficial venous outflow and pierces the superficial layer of the deep temporal fascia and empties into the middle temporal vein within the intermediate temporal fat pad. This is a low-flow system, and this vein can easily tamponade with excessive probe pressure. **(b, c)** Images obtained using an 18 MHz probe in vertical position on temple showing the sentinel vein piercing the superficial layer of the deep temporal fascia to enter the intermediate temporal fat pad (upper image). Lower image shows the middle temporal vein within the intermediate temporal fat confirmed by spectral doppler. The sentinel vein feeds into the middle temporal vein which then feeds into the internal jugular vein.

Key Point

The deep injection on bone technique had the greatest influence on improving the temporal volume (25.0%), the temporal crest (33.3%), and the lateral orbital rim visibility (31.0%) scales but had no effects in other facial regions. The interfascial injection technique revealed good effects on improving temporal hollowing (23.3%) but had an even greater effect on the crow's feet (26.8%) and on the position of the eyebrow (33.3%). The subdermal injection technique had its greatest effects in the lower face by improving the contour of the jawline (26.8%) followed by the improvement of the lower cheek fullness scale (14.3%).

If overall effect was reviewed, the interfascial plane injection created the most change to the face, with the subdermal (superficial fat pad) injection giving the least change.

A fourth plane of injection has been proposed and was recently described by Dr. Chris Surek. It involves ultrasound-guided injections into the intermediate temporal fat pad. Experience with ultrasound is required to avoid direct injection into the middle temporal vein (pulmonary embolus and death are rare complications). It seems to be a logical injection target to replace lost volume due to the aging fat loss (▶ Fig. 2.21, ▶ Fig. 2.22, ▶ Fig. 2.23, ▶ Fig. 2.24, ▶ Fig. 2.25, ▶ Fig. 2.26).

2.5 Ultrasound of the Forehead and Glabella

2.5.1 Supraorbital Artery Anatomy and Depth Transitions

The supraorbital artery is a branch of the ophthalmic artery which exits through either a supraorbital notch or foramen about 2.4 cm from the midline. It runs superiorly along the periosteum of the frontal bone for the first 13-14 mm of the forehead. At this point, it transitions into a more superficial plane, first intermuscular and in the subcutaneous plane. There are often communications between the anterior branch of the superficial temporal artery as well as the supratrochlear artery (▶ Fig. 2.27, ▶ Fig. 2.28, ▶ Fig. 2.29, ▶ Fig. 2.30).

2.5.2 Supratrochlear Artery Anatomy and Depth Transitions

The supratrochlear artery is a terminal branch of the ophthalmic artery and exits via a foramen or notch approximately 1.4 cm lateral to the midline. As it traverses over the superior orbital rim it lays deep to the corrugator supercilii. It will pierce the corrugator and run deep to the orbicularis oculi and then the frontalis along the periosteurm. At a distance of 14 mm above the orbital rim, the artery transitions more superficially, initially intramuscular and then in the subcutaneous plane. The supratrochlear artery is the most direct artery that can communicate with the ophthalmic artery which is pertinent in cases of filler associated blindness. The smallest volume of the STA from the orbital rim to the ophthalmic artery is 0.04 mL in a study of 12 arteries. This led many to recommend boluses near the eye should be less than 0.025 mL. (▶ Fig. 2.31, ▶ Fig. 2.32, ▶ Fig. 2.33, ▶ Fig. 2.34, ▶ Fig. 2.35)

There are communications of the supratrochlear artery with the supratrochlear of the opposite side, as well as the supraorbital and anterior branch of the superficial temporal artery.

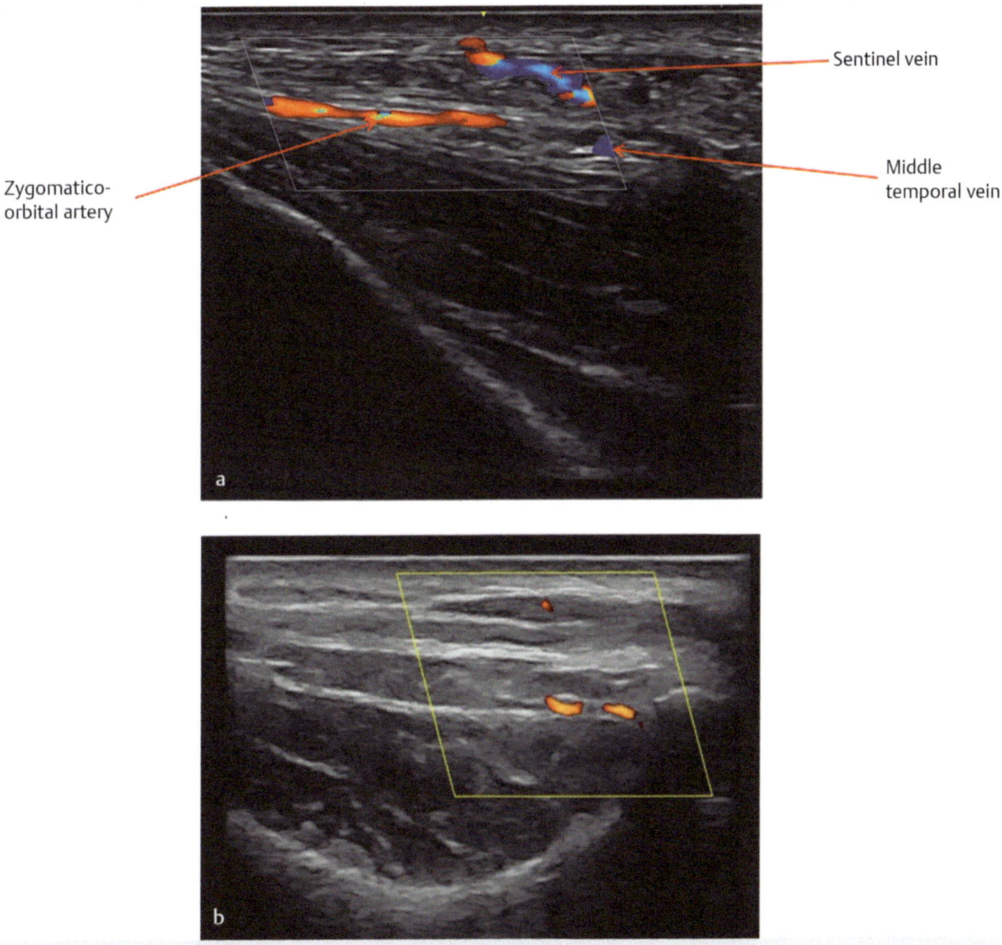

Fig. 2.16 **(a)** This color duplex image was obtained using a vertical 18-MHz probe. The sentinel vein is seen going from the superficial fat to emptying into the middle temporal vein, which lies within the intermediate temporal fat pad. The zygomatico-orbital artery is found just deep to the superficial layer of the deep temporal fascia. Its position is highly variable and can also be found in the interfascial plane. There are documented cases of pulmonary embolus and death related to filler injection into the middle temporal vein. **(b)** 20 MHz handheld probe in horizontal position showing a deep zygomatico-orbital artery laying in the intermediate temporal fat and piercing the deep layer of the deep temporal fascia.

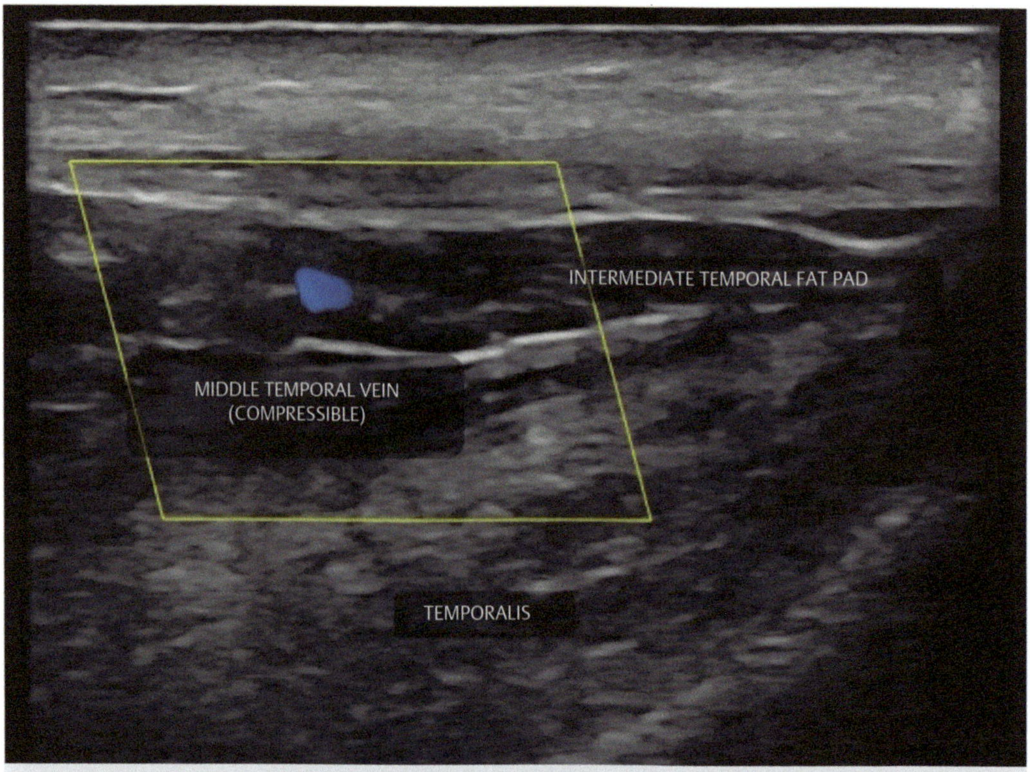

Fig. 2.17 Image obtained using a vertical 20-MHz probe showing the middle temporal vein within the intermediate temporal fat pad. This vessel in compressible confirming it is a vein.

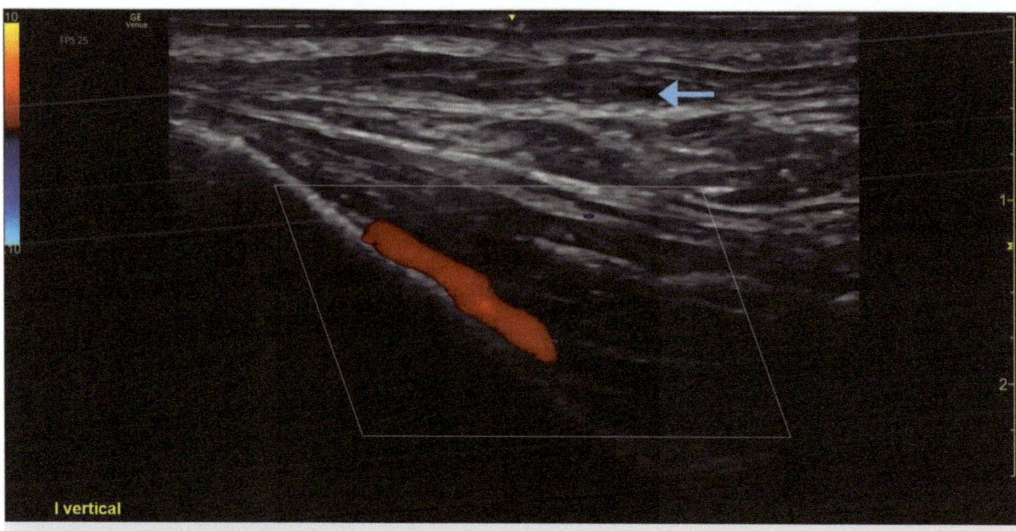

Fig. 2.18 Color Doppler image obtained using slightly off vertical position, parallel to the orbital rim, using a 12-MHz probe. There are two deep temporal arteries (anterior and posterior) that run along the temporal bone in a vertical position. The branching pattern and position are highly variable, and there is no safe injection location for the deep periosteal injection These arteries originate from the internal maxillary artery and therefore communicate with the internal carotid system. To visualize the deep temporal arteries (anterior and posterior), sometimes a 12-MHz probe is recommended versus an 18- or 20-MHz probe. Hyaluronic acid (HA) filler is also found within the interfascial plane (blue arrow).

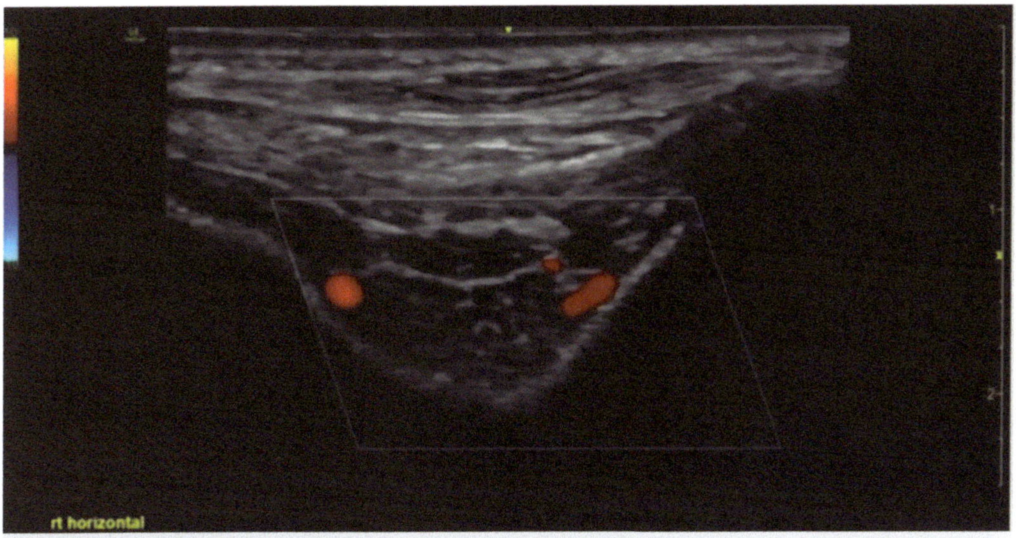

Fig. 2.19 Color Doppler image obtained using a horizontal 12-MHz probe. The anterior and posterior deep temporal arteries are visualized lying deep in temporal fossa, seen in cross section.

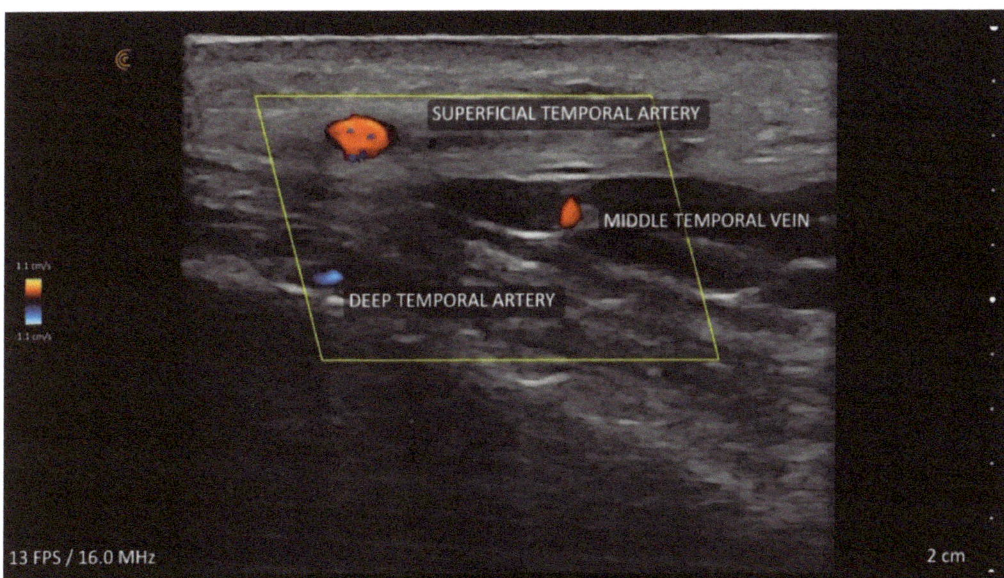

Fig. 2.20 Color Doppler image obtained using a vertical 20-MHz probe showing the relationship between the anterior branch of the superficial temporal artery (STA), the middle temporal vein, and the anterior branch of the deep temporal artery.

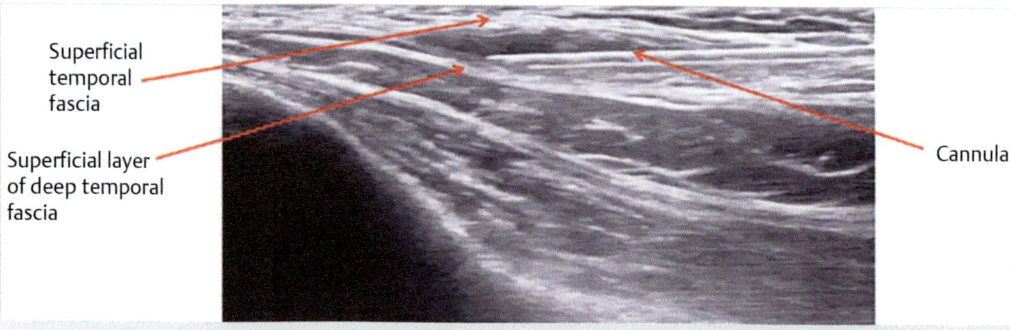

Fig. 2.21 20 MHz vertical probe showing a microcannula injecting filler in the interfascial plane. Anechoic HA filler is seen near tip of cannula.

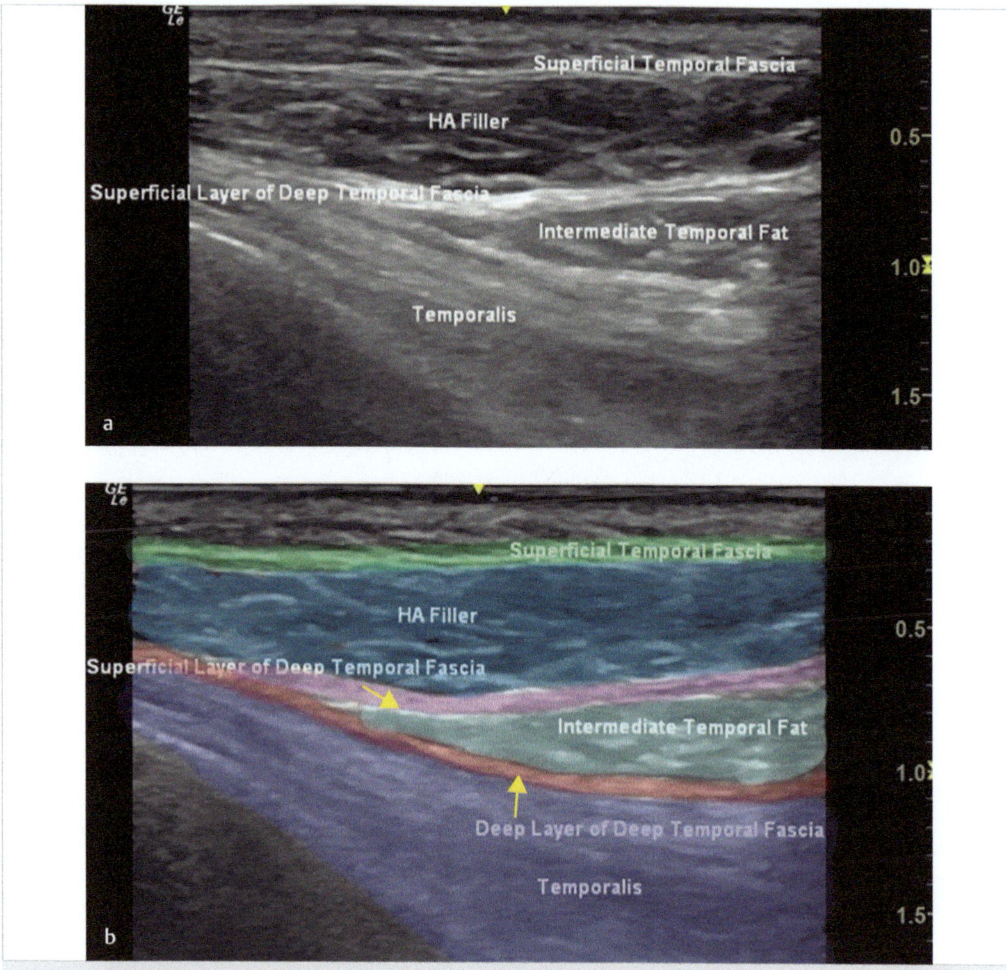

Fig. 2.22 **(a, b)** Image obtained using an 18-MHz probe in vertical position after hyaluronic acid injection in interfascial plane. The filler is location between the superficial musculoaponeurotic system (SMAS) (superficial temporal fascia) and the superficial layer of the deep temporal fascia. Hyaluronic acid (HA) filler in the interfascial plane can create a significant volume change in the temple.

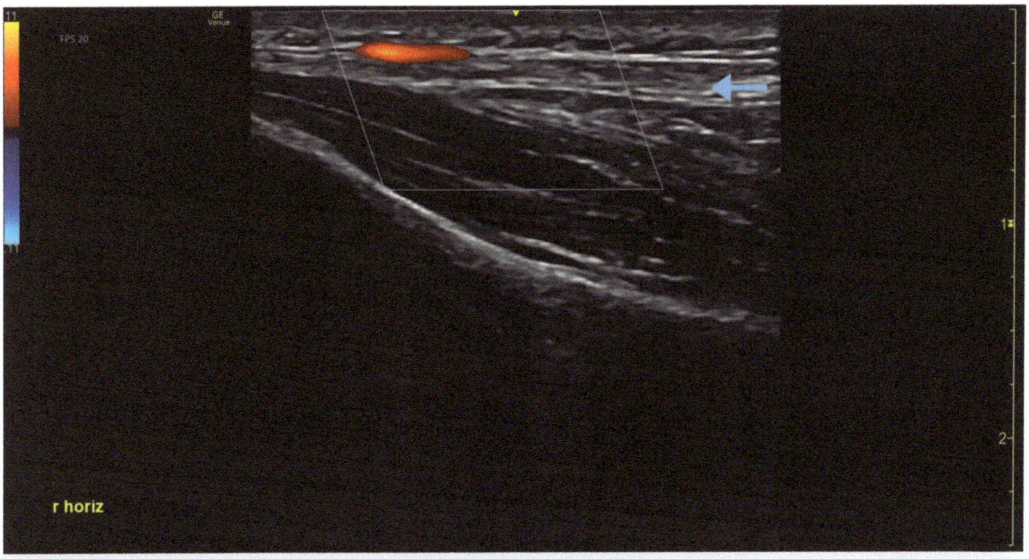

Fig. 2.23 Color Duplex image obtained using an 18-MHz horizontal probe showing the anterior branch of the superficial temporal fascia in the superficial musculoaponeurotic system (SMAS) layer with hyaluronic acid filler within the interfascial plane (blue arrow). Note the clear distinction between the SMAS and the superficial layer of the deep temporal fascia.

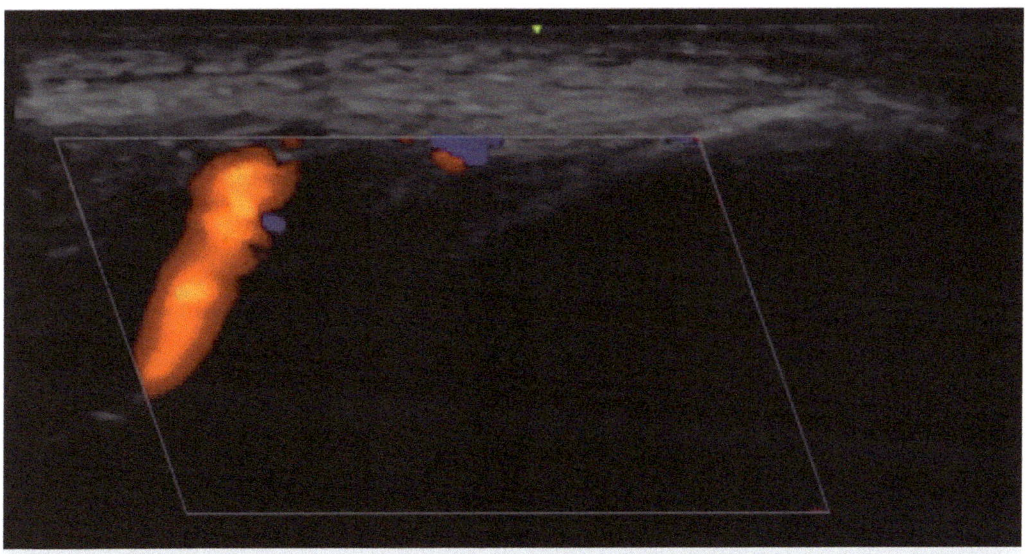

Fig. 2.24 12 MHz probe showing the zygomaticotemporal artery. This artery is distinct from the deep temporal artery because it doesn't lie along the temporal bone but it does communicate with it. It arises from the lacrimal artery and exits the zygomaticotemporal foramen on the back surface of the zygomatic bone.

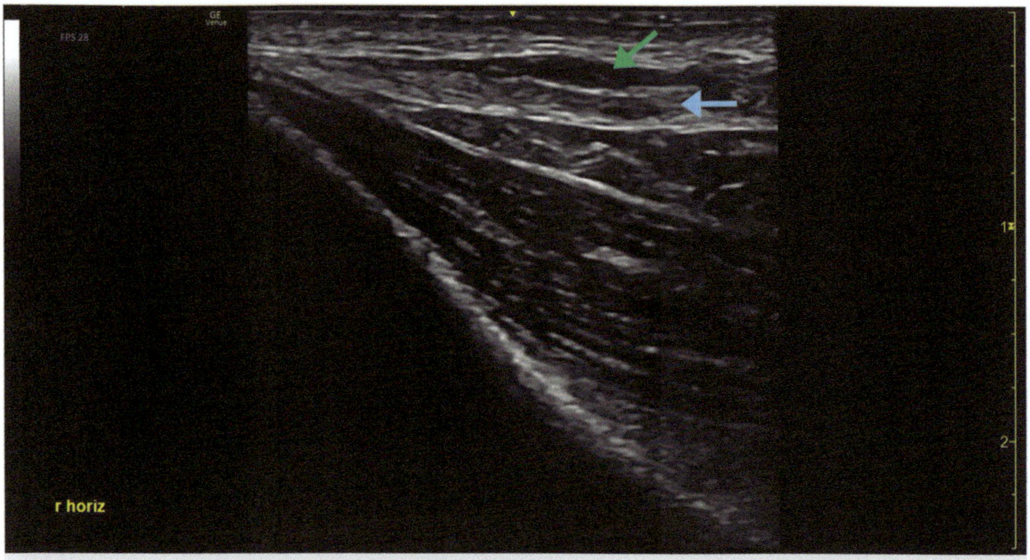

Fig. 2.25 Image obtained using an 18-MHz probe in vertical position. Hyaluronic acid (HA) filler is within the superficial musculoaponeurotic system (SMAS) (green arrow). It is postulated that a filler within a fascial layer is at more risk to form nodules or granulomas. Interfascial plane is show with blue arrow.

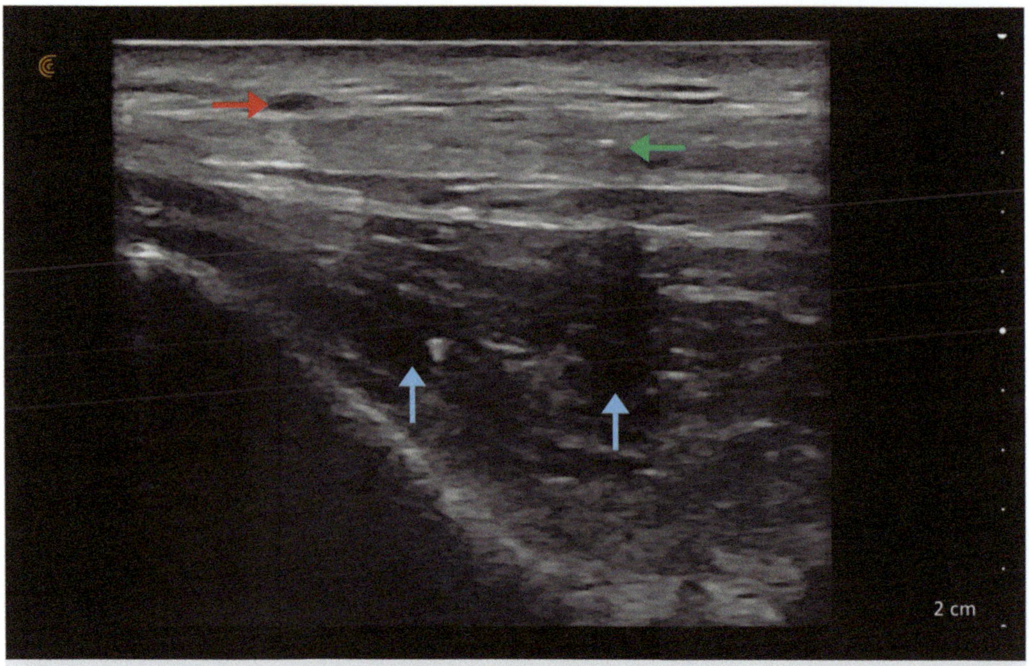

Fig. 2.26 Image obtained using a 20-MHz handheld probe in vertical position, immediately after injection of hyaluronic acid (HA) on periosteum of temple (blue arrows) and interfascial plane injection of poly-l-lactic acid (PLLA) (green arrow). Note that the HA spreads within the temporalis muscle. Also note the cross section of the anterior branch of the superficial temporal artery in upper left part of the image with the superficial musculoaponeurotic system (SMAS) layer (red arrow).

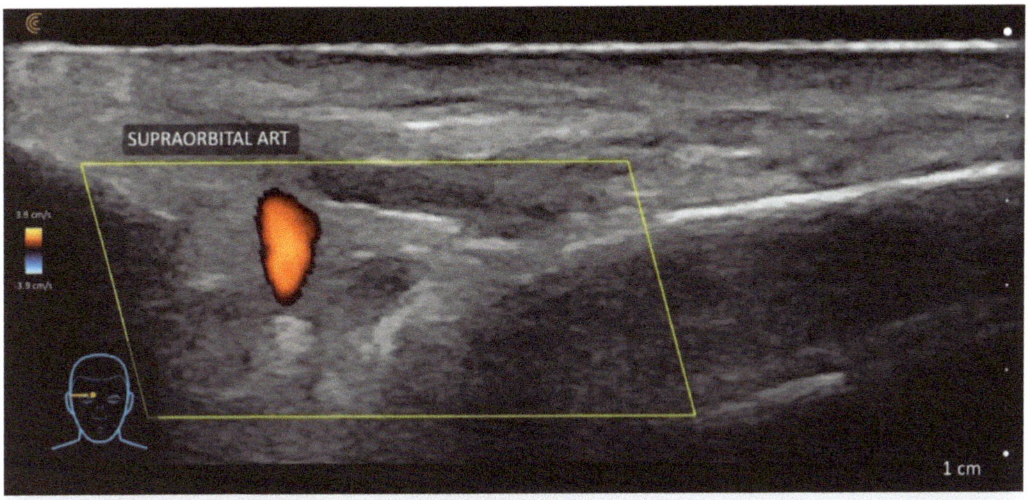

Fig. 2.27 Image obtained using a 20-MHz probe in horizontal position. Supraorbital artery is seen exiting the supraorbital notch. It lies deep in this position and can be a single vessel or multiple vessels. It has a medium flow velocity.

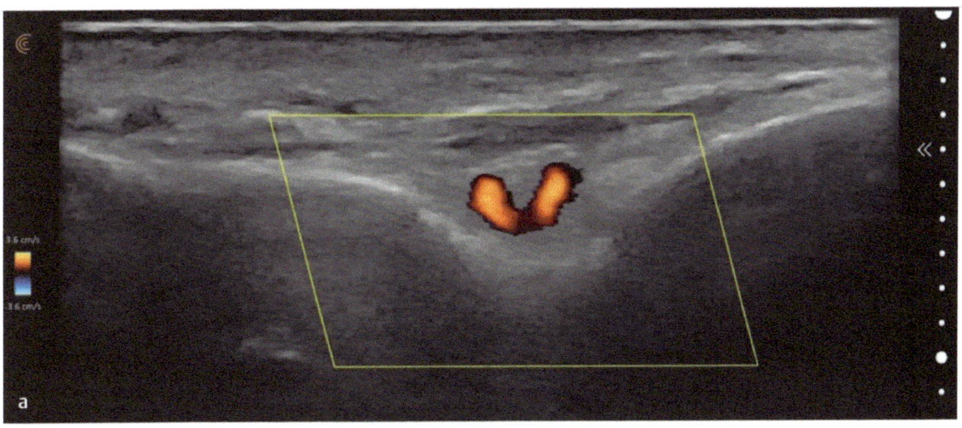

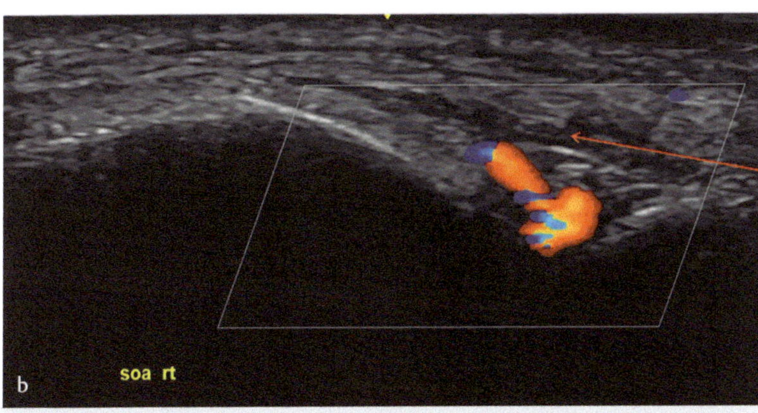

Orbicularis oculi muscle

Fig. 2.28 **(a)** Image obtained using a 20-MHz handheld probe. The supraorbital artery is emerging from the supraorbital notch in a double vessel variation. **(b)** Image obtained with an 18 MHz probe in horizontal position showing the supraorbital artery emerging from its notch. At this point, it is below the orbicularis oculi muscle.

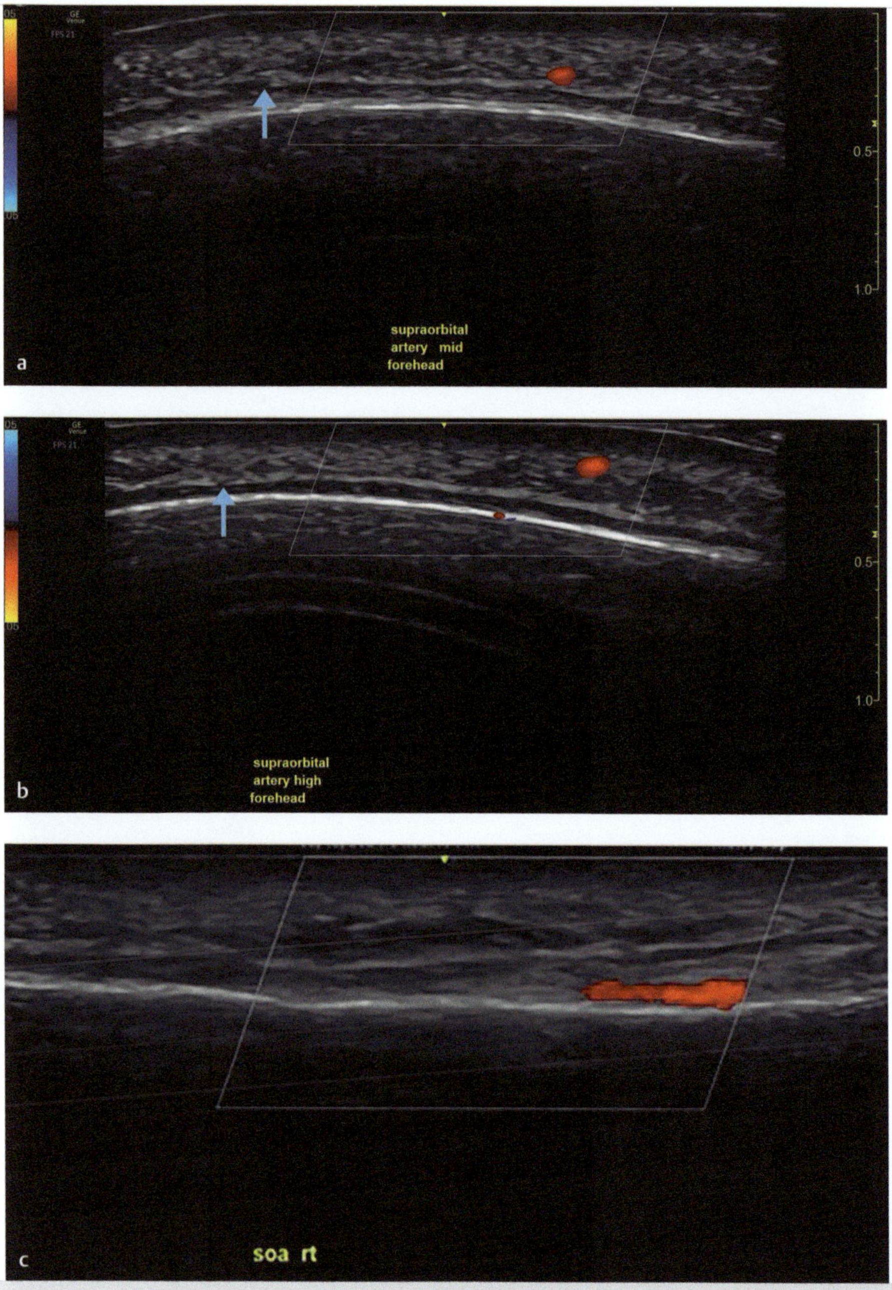

Fig. 2.29 **(a, b)** Images obtained using an 18-MHz probe in horizontal position. Note the changes in the depth (from deep to more superficial) of the supraorbital artery as it travels more superior. The frontalis muscle is hypoechoic and marked with blue arrow. The artery remains submuscular for the first 15 mm from the orbital rim and then transitions to intramuscular in the middle third of the forehead, eventually transitioning to subcutaneous in the upper third of the forehead. **(c, d)** 18 MHz vertical probe showing the supraorbital artery (SOA) laying along the periosteum for the initial ~ 15 mm and then transitioning through the frontalis muscle at 15–20 mm above the orbital rim to a more superficial position. The hypoechoic linear structure running horizontally is the frontalis muscle.

(Continued)

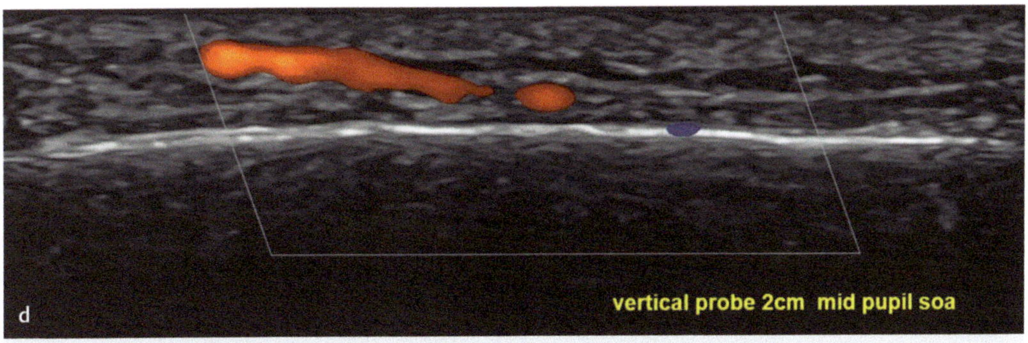

Fig. 2.29 (*Continued*) (d)

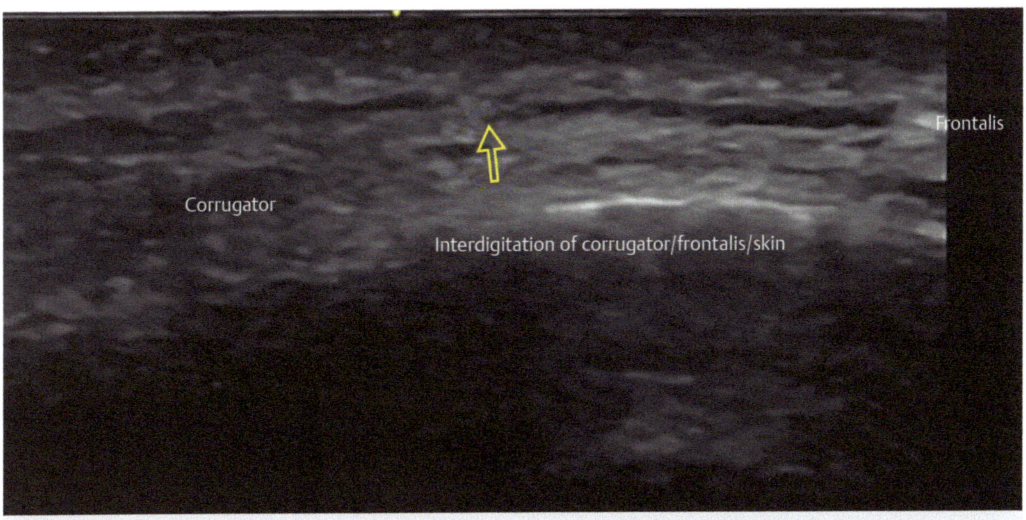

Fig. 2.30 Image taken with the 18 MHz probe in horizontal position. The lateral corrugator interdigitates with the frontalis muscle and skin near the mid pupillary line. Arrow points to the point of interdigitation.

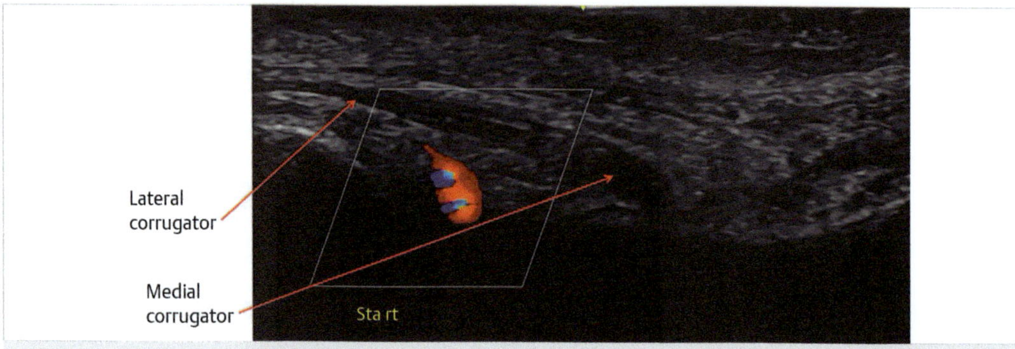

Fig. 2.31 Image obtained using an 18-MHz probe in horizontal position. The supratrochlear artery is seen deep along the bone as it emerges from the supratrochlear notch. Note its position below the corrugator supercilii muscle in this position. Also note the orientation of the corrugator with lateral corrugator muscle tail (left side of image) located more superficial than the medial corrugator muscle (right side of image).

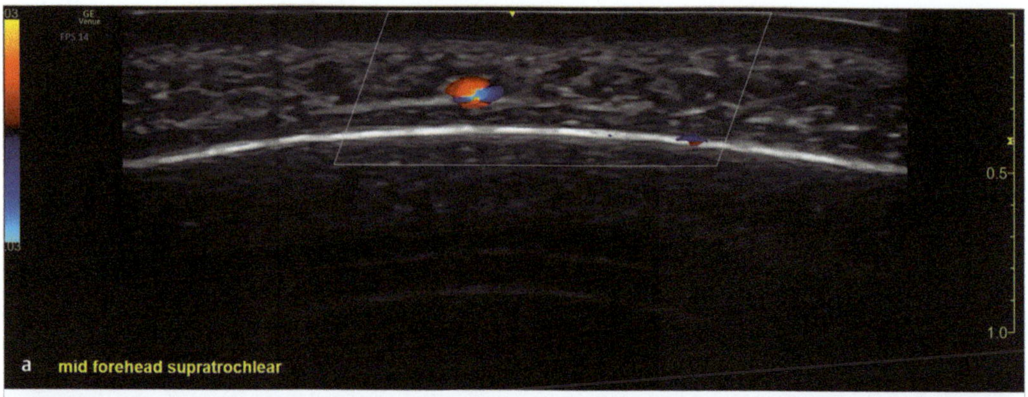

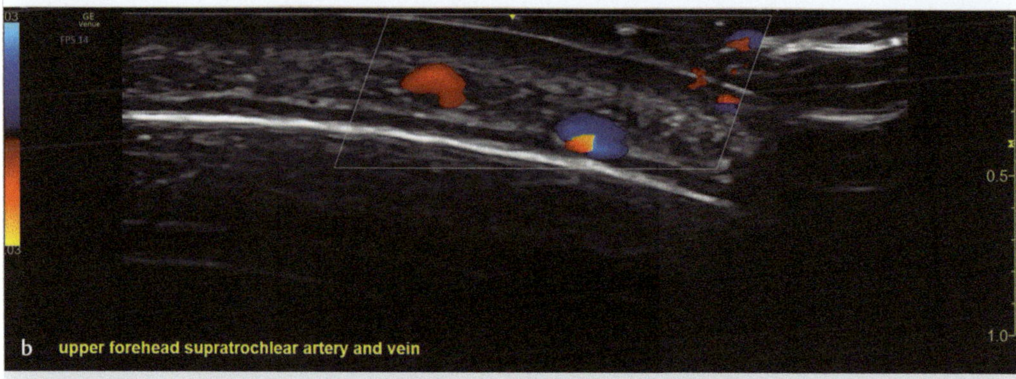

Fig. 2.32 **(a, b)** Images obtained using an 18-MHz horizontal probe with color Doppler. Similar to the supraorbital artery, the supratrochlear artery becomes more superficial as it travels up the forehead. A large vein (blue) is also seen in the lower image.

(Continued)

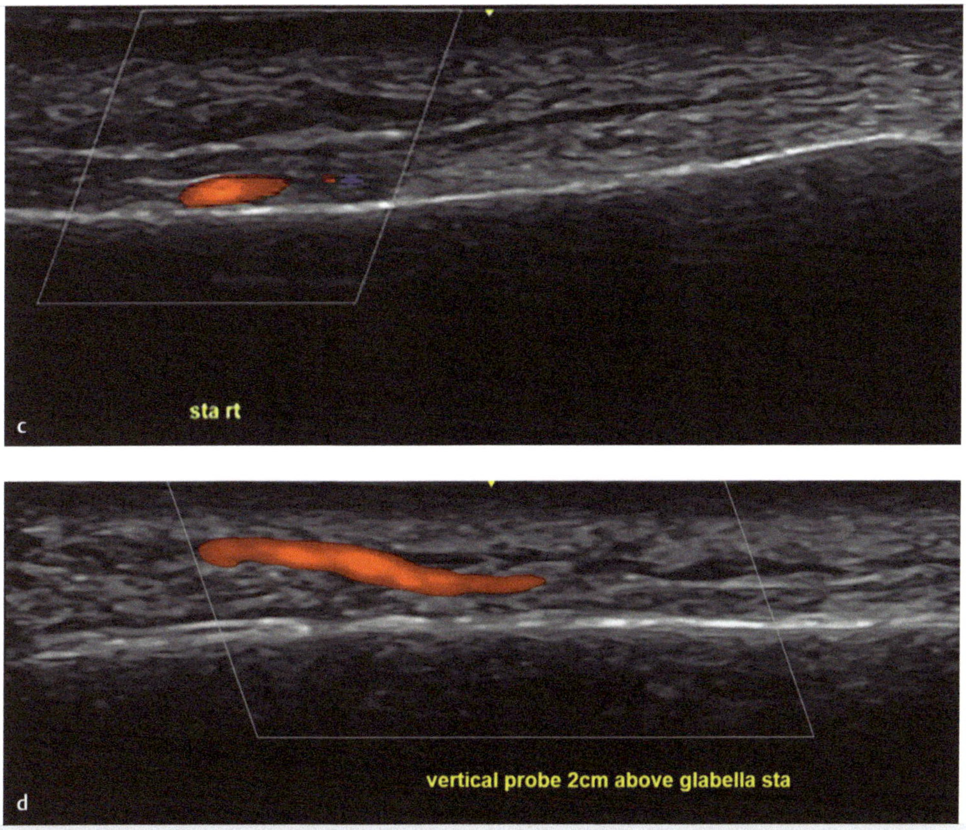

Fig. 2.32 (*Continued*) **(c, d)** 18 MHz vertical probe showing the supratrochlear artery (STA) laying along the periosteum for the initial ~ 14 mm and then transitioning through the frontalis muscle at ~ 14 mm above the orbital rim to a more superficial position. The hypoechoic linear structure running horizontally is the frontalis muscle.

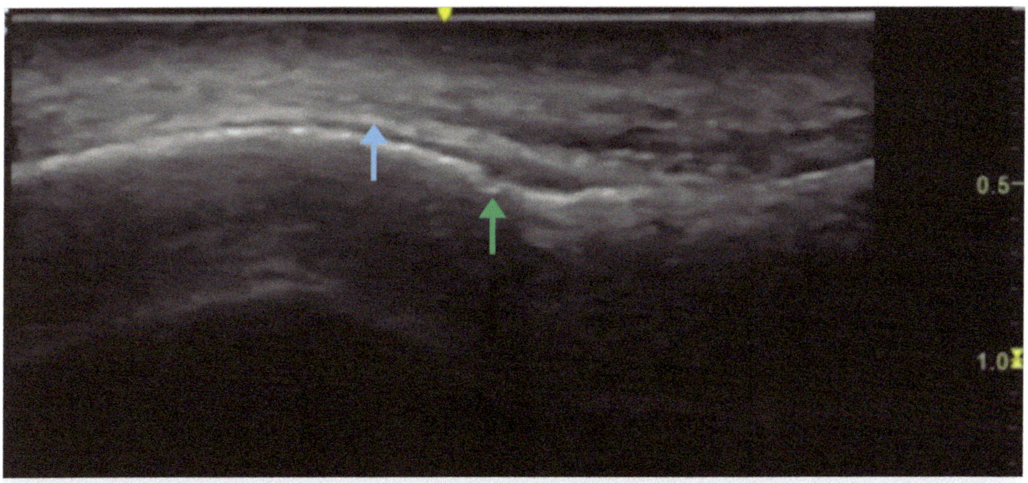

Fig. 2.33 Image obtained using an 18-MHz probe in vertical position. The procerus muscle (blue arrow) is arising from the nasal bone and inserting into the skin in glabellar area. The nasion (green arrow) is visualized and is the suture line between the nasal and frontal bones. The procerus origin from the bone can be seen to the right of the image and the interdigitation with the dermis on the left of the image.

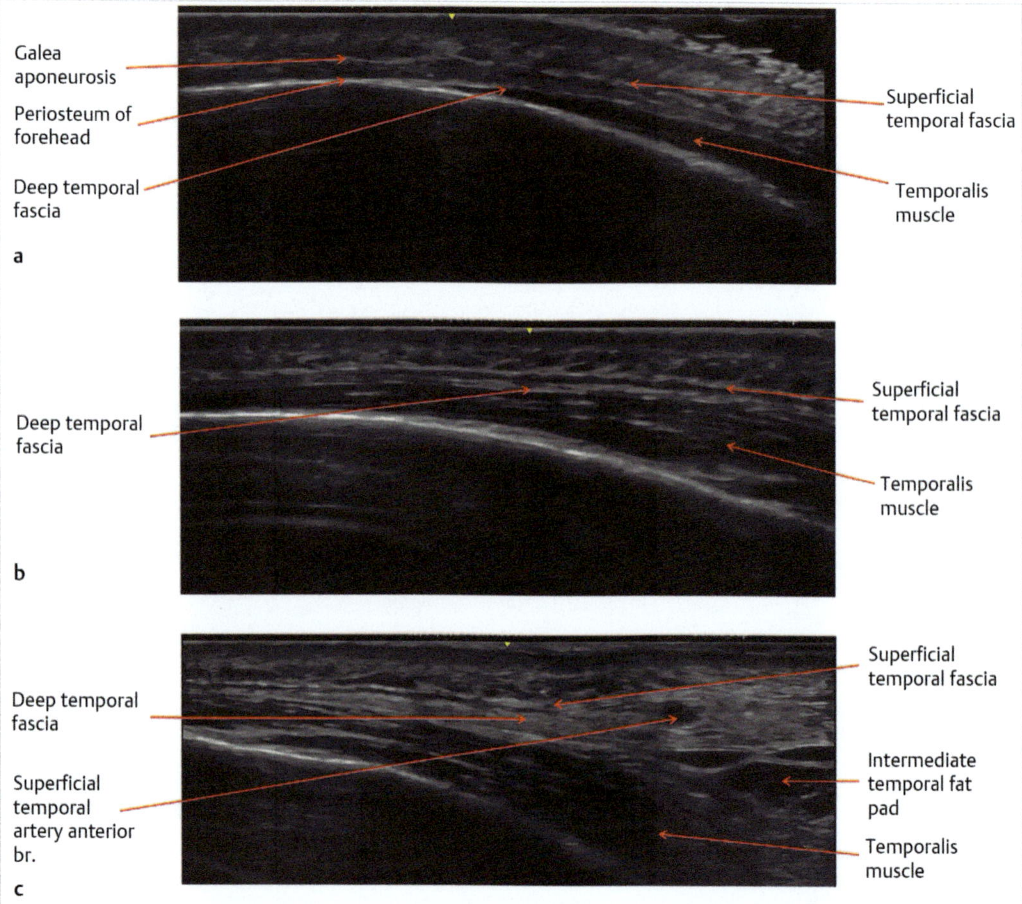

Fig. 2.34 (a–c) Images obtained using 20 MHz probe in vertical position from forehead to temple. The order of the images is superior to inferior. The periosteum of the forehead becomes the deep temporal fascia as it goes laterally. The galea aponeurosis becomes the superficial temporal fascia (SMAS) as it goes laterally. The deep temporal fascia thickens and then splits into a superficial and deep layer, with the intermediate temporal fat pad lying between these two layers. The superficial temporal artery, anterior branch, is enveloped by the superficial temporal fascia. The temporalis muscle is covered superficially by the deep layer of the deep temporal fascia. Note that there is no periosteum along the temporal bone which is covered by the temporalis muscle. Also note that the plane between the superficial and deep temporal fascia (interfascial plane) is not visualized on lower image and this is commonly the case because these two layers are tightly opposed to each other and the interfascial plane or upper temporal space is a potential space.

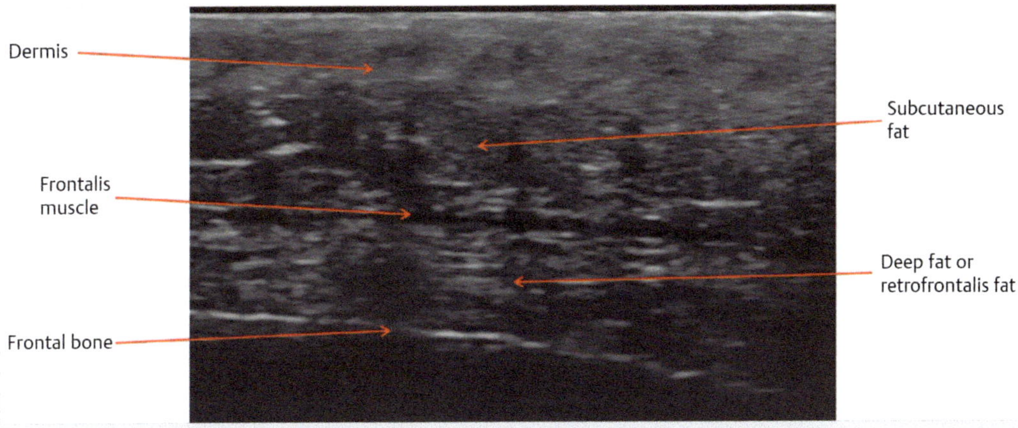

Fig. 2.35 Image obtained with a 70 MHz probe in a horizontal position 2 cm above orbital rim in paramedian position. The amount of deep fat decreases and then ceases as you go superiorly towards hairline. The muscle is covered superficial by the suprafrontalis fascia and deep by the subfrontalis fascia. The two fascia and the muscle combine to form the galea aponeurosis. Above the orbital rim, the deep fat is called the ROOF (retro-orbicularis oculi fat). The authors (SW and CS) recommended plane of injection is below the galea at least 15 mm above the orbital rim using cannula.

Suggested Readings

Beleznay K, Carruthers JDA, Humphrey S, Carruthers A, Jones D. Update on avoiding and treating blindness from fillers: a recent review of the world literature. Aesthet Surg J. 2019; 39 (6):662–674

Bozikov K, Shaw-Dunn J, Soutar DS, Arnez ZM. Arterial anatomy of the lateral orbital and cheek region and arterial supply to the "peri-zygomatic perforator arteries" flap. Surg Radiol Anat. 2008 ;30(1):17-22

Casabona G, Frank K, Moellhoff N, et al. Full-face effects of temporal volumizing and temporal lifting techniques. J Cosmet Dermatol. 2020; 19(11):2830–2837

Correa BJ, Weathers WM, Wolfswinkel EM, Thornton JF. The forehead flap: the gold standard of nasal soft tissue reconstruction. Semin Plast Surg. 2013; 27(2):96–103. Thieme

Cotofana S, Velthuis PJ, Alfertshofer M, Frank K, Bertucci V, Beleznay K, Swift A, Gavril DL, Lachman N, Schelke L. The change of plane of the supratrochlear and supraorbital arteries in the forehead—an ultrasound-based investigation. Aesthet Surg J. 2021; 41(11): NP1589-NP1598

Cotofana S, Gaete A, Hernandez CA, et al. The six different injection techniques for the temple relevant for soft tissue filler augmentation procedures—clinical anatomy and danger zones. J Cosmet Dermatol. 2020; 19(7):1570–1579

Kareem ZM, Muthana A, Hassan SF, et al. Supraorbital artery: Anatomical variations and neurosurgical applications. Surg Neurol Int. 2023;14:318

Khan TT, Colon-Acevedo B, Mettu P, DeLorenzi C, Woodward JA. An anatomical analysis of the supratrochlear artery: considerations in facial filler injections and preventing vision loss. Aesthet Surg J. 2017; 37(2):203–208

Lamb J, Surek C. Facial Volumization: An Anatomic Approach. 1st ed. New York, NY: Thieme Medical Publishers; 2017

Moss CJ, Mendelson BC, Taylor GI. Surgical anatomy of the ligamentous attachments in the temple and periorbital regions. Plast Reconstr Surg. 2000; 105(4):1475–1490, discussion 1491–1498

Mendelson B, Wong CH. Anatomy of the aging face. In: Neligan PC, ed. Plastic Surgery. Philadelphia, PA: Elsevier; 2013:78-92

Nikolis A, Enright KM, Troupis T, et al. Topography of the deep temporal arteries and implications for performing safe aesthetic injections. J Cosmet Dermatol. 2022; 21(2):608–614

O'Brien JX, Ashton MW, Rozen WM, Ross R, Mendelson BC. New perspectives on the surgical anatomy and nomenclature of the temporal region: literature review and dissection study. Plast Reconstr Surg. 2013; 131(3):510–522. Discussion by D. Knize on 523–525

Pankratz J, Baer J, Mayer C, et al. Depth transitions of the frontal branch of the facial nerve: implications in SMAS rhytidectomy. JPRAS Open. 2020; 26:101–108

Surek C. Facial anatomy for filler injection: the superficial musculoaponeurotic system (SMAS) is not just for facelifting. Clin Plast Surg 2019; 46(4):603-612

Surek CC. A new target for temple volumization? An anatomical and ultrasound-guided study of the intermediate temporal fat pad. Aesthet Surg J. 2021; 41(12):1339–1343

Vaca EE, Purnell CA, Gosain AK, Alghoul MS. Postoperative temporal hollowing: Is there a surgical approach that prevents this complication? A systematic review and anatomic illustration. J Plast Reconstr Aesthet Surg. 2017; 70(3):401–415

Walker L, Cetto R. Facial Ageing and Injection Anatomy. 1st ed. UK Book Publishing; 2021

Zito PM, Chauhan PR. Anatomy, Head and Neck, Supratrochlear. 2023 Jul 24. In: StatPearls [Internet]. Treasure Island (FL): StatPearls Publishing; 2024

Chapter 3

Layered Anatomy of the Middle Face

3

3 Layered Anatomy of the Middle Face

Abstract
The midface contains the prezygomatic space, suborbicularis oculi fat (SOOF), deep pyriform space, and deep medial/lateral cheek fat. With age volume is lost in the SOOF and deep cheek fat along with bony resorption in the maxilla and pyriform fossa. This chapter will describe the three-dimensional layering of the midface, outlining possible targets for injection procedures as well as the vascular anatomy of this region relevant to the clinical injector. Anatomical descriptions are then complemented by detailed ultrasound visuals and technique pearls when imaging the midface anatomy.

Keywords: Pre-zygomatic space, deep pyriform space, deep medial cheek fat, deep lateral cheek fat, suborbicularis oculi fat (SOOF), orbital retaining ligament, zygomaticocutaneous retaining ligament, angular artery, angular vein, levator labii superioris muscle, nasolabial fold, nasolabial fat compartment, nasolabial fold, lateral nasal artery, columellar artery, dorsal nasal artery, dorsal nasal vein

3.1 Nose

The framework of the nose is formed by the nasal bones superiorly and the upper and lower lateral cartilages inferiorly. There is a robust vascular network supplying the soft tissue of the nose including the columellar, and lateral nasal and dorsal nasal vessels. The nasal superficial musculoaponeurotic system (SMAS) is on average 0.6 mm in deep to the skin surface. The nasal vasculature most commonly travels within the nasal SMAS. Dermal filler injections should be targeted deep to the nasal SMAS on the periosteum or perichondrium. The dorsal nasal vessels have a direct vascular connection to the ophthalmic vasculature. The nose is the most common location of filler injection vision compromise (▶ Fig. 3.1).

3.2 Nasolabial Fold

The nasolabial fold demarcates a transition zone between the cheek and perioral aesthetic subunits. The fold is created by septations from the lip elevator muscles to the skin. Descent of the nasolabial fat pad with age leads to a tissue bulging over the fold and a deepening shadow within the fold. Bone loss in the pyriform aperture contributes to the deepening of the nasolabial fold with age (▶ Fig. 3.2).

3.3 Lateral Cheek

The zygomatic arch forms the lateral boundary of the cheek. The arch traverses medially until it transitions to the body of the zygoma. This transition is a palpable bony step-off and corresponds with the location of the main zygomatic retaining ligament and origin of the zygomaticus major muscle. Two key vascular structures related to the zygomatic arch are the middle temporal vein which is superior and deep to the arch and the transverse facial artery (TFA) which traverses parallel to the arch just below the inferior border of the bone. The TFA divides into fascial and muscular branches. The fascial branch commonly sends a transzygomatic branch that travels over the periosteum of the arch often in the middle third of the arch. These transzygomatic branches may create a vascular pathway between the internal carotid and external carotid artery systems. Injectors must be cognizant of this vascular relationship when preforming injection procedures along the zygomatic arch.

3.4 Anterior Upper Midface

The bony components of the upper midface include the orbital rim, body of zygoma, and maxilla. The maxilla bone is more susceptible to age-related bony resorption compared to the zygoma. The prezygomatic space is a potential gliding space deep to the orbicularis oculi muscle residing on the body of the zygoma. The space has been established as a good injection target for midface volumization. The deep fat compartment of the upper midface is the suborbicularis oculi fat (SOOF) compartment. Surface volumetric studies have shown significant topographic changes following volumization of the SOOF compared to other deep fat compartments in the face. This likely relates to the role of the retaining ligaments in this region limiting superior and inferior migration of the product, and forcing injection product to project outward and create enhanced cheek volume (▶ Fig. 3.3).

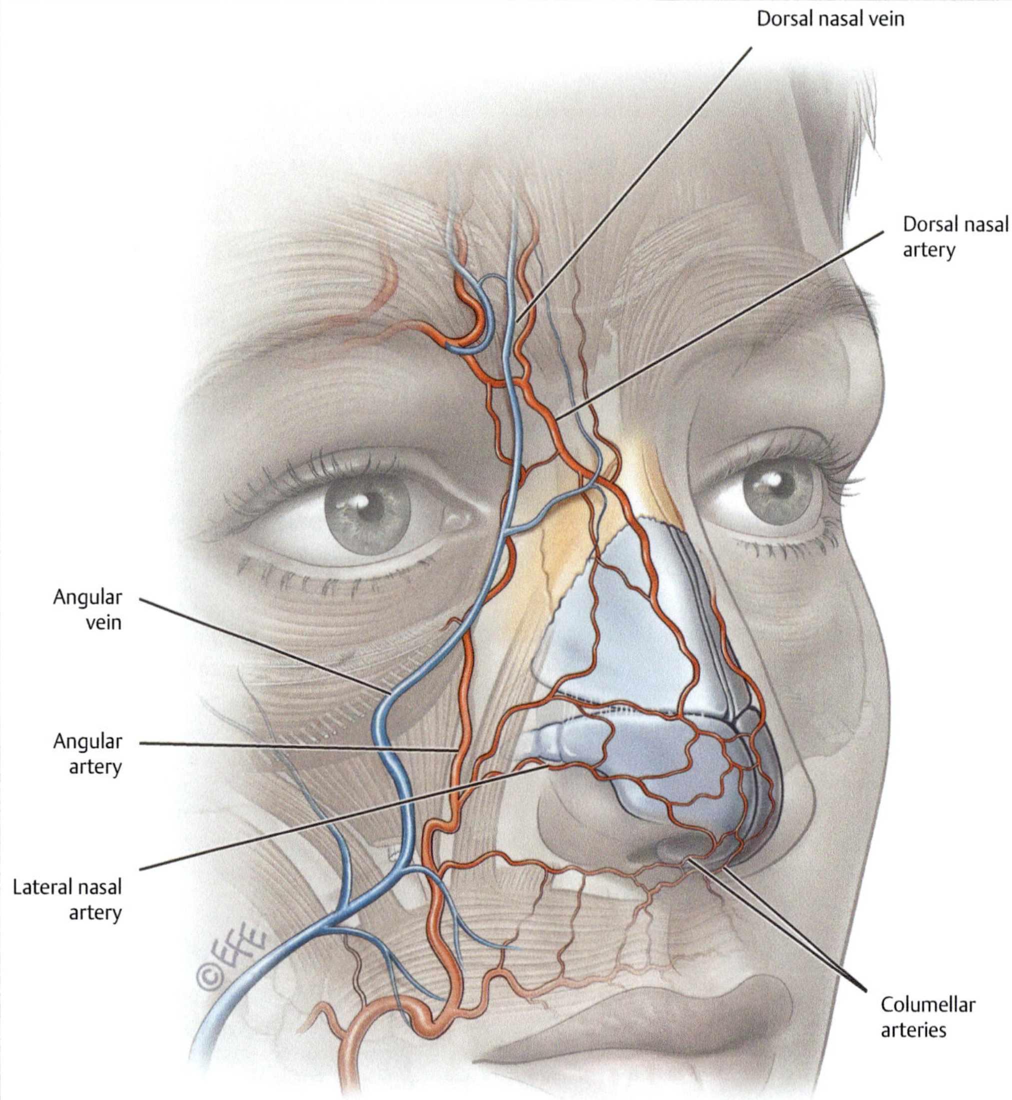

Fig. 3.1 Anatomic illustration of the nasal vasculature. The nasal blood supply consists of the columellar artery, lateral nasal artery, and dorsal nasal artery. © Dr. Levent Efe, CMI.

The retaining ligament boundaries of the prezygomatic space are the orbital retaining ligament (ORL) and the zygomaticocutaneous ligaments (ZCL) respectively. At the lateral boundary of the space is the main zygomatic retaining ligament located at the junction of the zygomatic arch and body and corresponds with the muscular origin of the zygomaticus major muscle. The zygomatic ligament is biomechanically the stiffest ligament in the face. The ORL is the superior boundary and separates the prezygomatic space from the preseptal space of the lower eyelid. The ORL is the second stiffest ligament biomechanically in the face. The ZCL are the inferior boundary of the space and separate the prezygomatic space from the deep medial cheek fat (DMCF) compartments and buccal fat. The ORL and ZCL are both considered osseocutaneous or "true" facial retaining ligaments because they travel from bone all

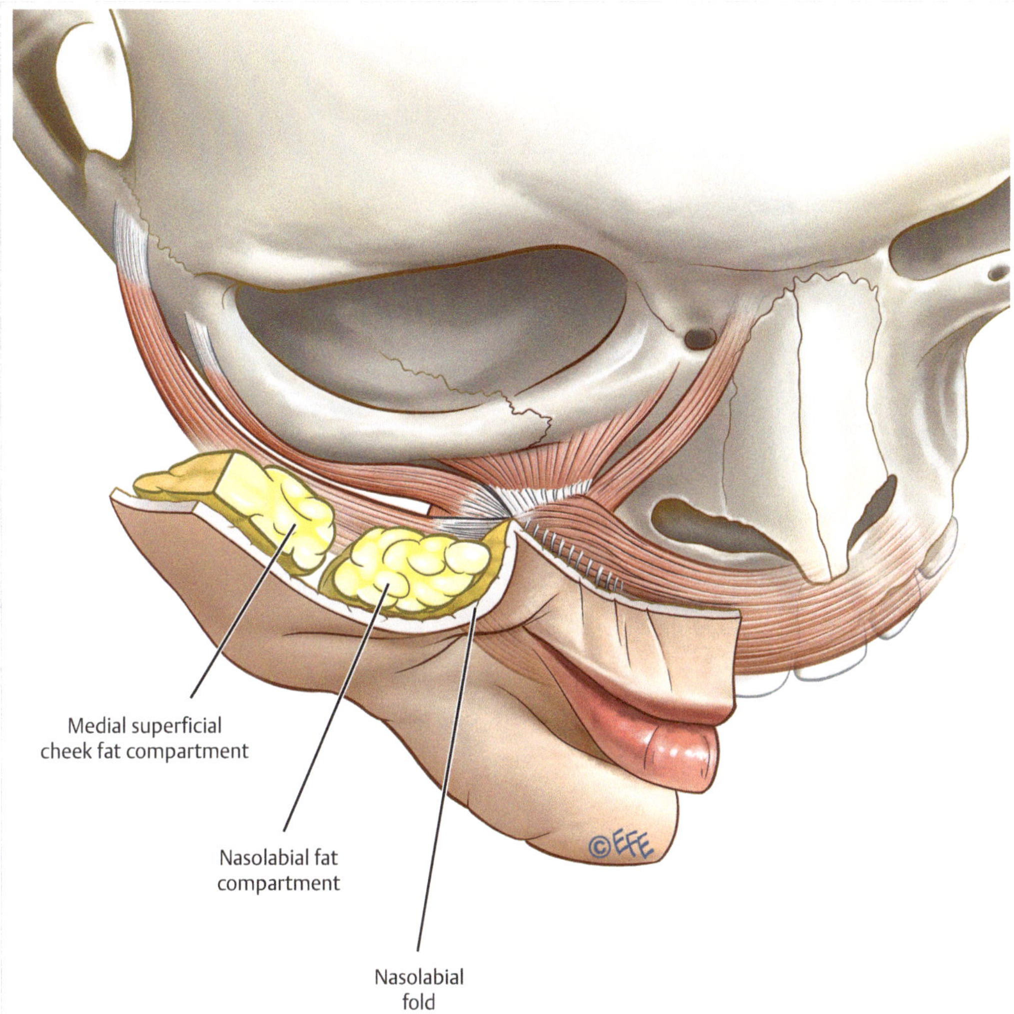

Fig. 3.2 Anatomic illustration of the nasolabial fold (NLF). The NLF is formed by septations from the lip elevator muscles to the skin. During the aging process, the nasolabial fat compartment descends creating a volume overhang and exaggeration of the nasolabial fold shadowing. © Dr. Levent Efe, CMI.

the way to the skin. Therefore, the ligaments begin on periosteum, traverse through the orbicularis oculi muscle, and insert onto the dermis of the skin to create the commonly known surface topography of the lid–cheek junction (ORL insertion) and nasojugal groove (ZCL insertion) (▶ Fig. 3.4).

In regard to facial vasculature, the most common pathway of the angular artery and vein is medial to the ZCL and ORL. The angular vein travels on the undersurface the ZCL as it traverses to the tear trough. A known aberrant branch of the angular artery runs within the midpupillary line but in the subcutaneous plane. The infraorbital neurovascular bundle is located inferior and medial to ZCL. The infraorbital foramen is located 6.3 to 10.9 cm inferior to the orbital rim between the midpupillary line and a vertical line from the medial corneal limbus. The supraorbital and infraorbital foramen have been found in the same vertical plane in 50% of cases. Therefore, clinical injections that stay within the confines of the ZCL and ORL avoid interaction with the most common pathways and variant pathways of the angular artery and vein as well as the infraorbital neurovascular bundle.

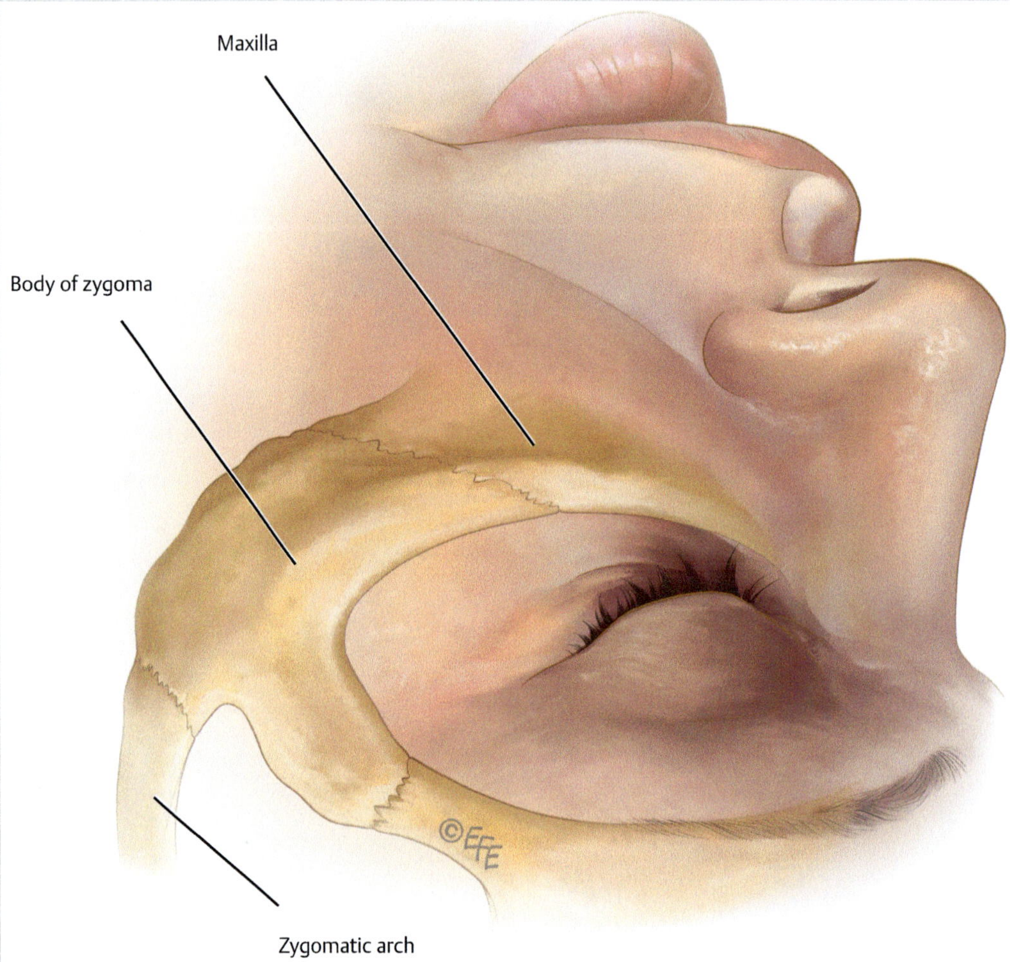

Fig. 3.3 Anatomic illustration of the bony architecture of the midface, which includes the zygomatic arch, body of zygoma, and maxilla. © Dr. Levent Efe, CMI.

Key Point

The prezygomatic space is a suitable target for cheek volumization and has distinct boundaries that can be readily palpated with a blunt tip cannula and/or identified under ultrasound examination. The most commonly pathways of the angular artery and vein are either superficial or medial to the prezygomatic space. The infraorbital neurovascular bundle is inferior and medial to the space. Therefore, injections targeted within the confines of the space may avoid interaction with these vascular structures and associated adverse events.

Additionally, consideration must be given to the lymphatic anatomy of the upper midface. There is one medial and two lateral lymphatic chains in the midface. Laterally, there is a superficial lateral lymphatic chain and a deep lateral lymphatic chain. The lymphatic chains originate in the lower eyelid and travel inferiorly. The deep lateral lymphatic chain courses deep to the orbicularis muscle and drains through the floor of the prezygomatic space, whereas the superficial lateral lymphatic chain travels superficial to the orbicularis muscle within the malar fat compartment. Clinically, disruption of the superficial lateral lymphatic chain can create an iatrogenic malar mound trapping fluid between the cutaneous insertions of the ORL and ZCL (▸ Fig. 3.5, ▸ Fig. 3.6, ▸ Fig. 3.7, ▸ Fig. 3.8).

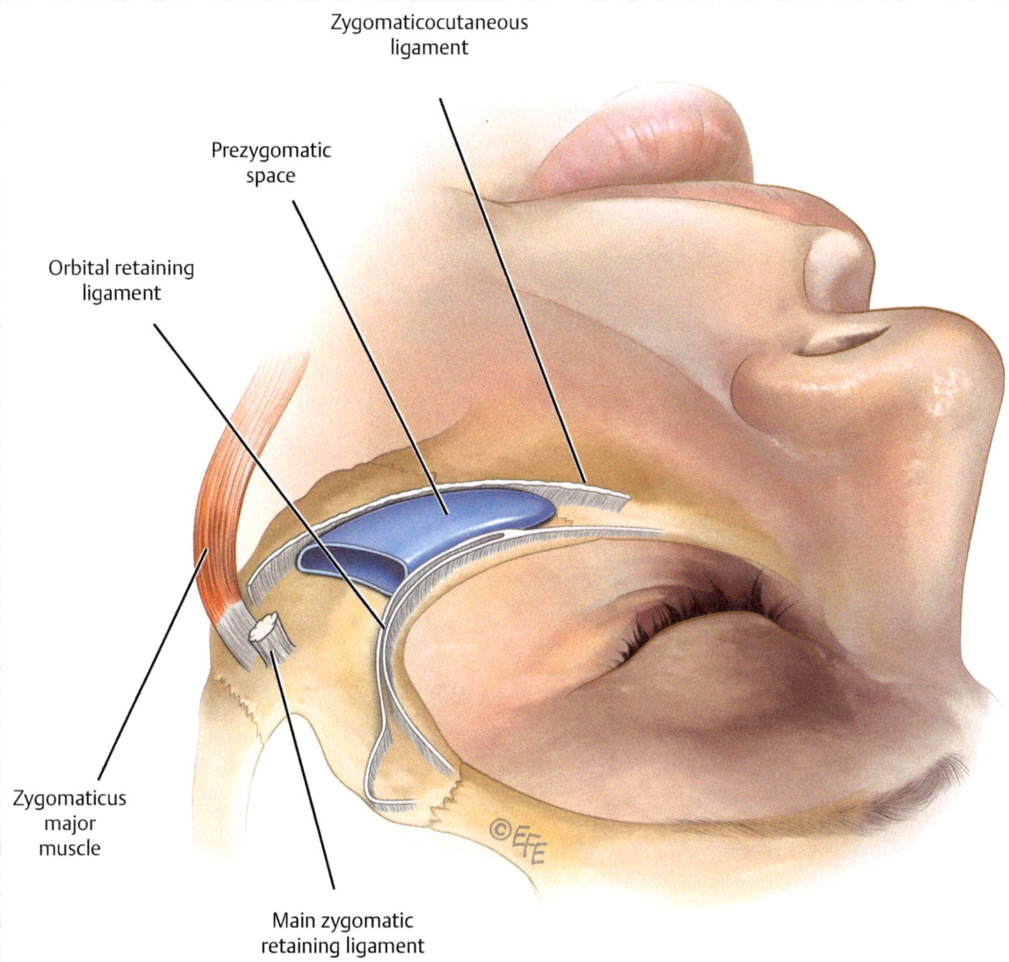

Fig. 3.4 Anatomic illustration of the sub-superficial musculoaponeurotic system (sub-SMAS) layer of the midface. The prezygomatic space is a gliding potential space deep to the orbicularis muscle. The superior boundary of the prezygomatic space is the orbital retaining ligament (ORL) and the inferior boundary is the zygomaticocutaneous ligaments (ZCL). The main zygomatic retaining ligament is located at the transition of the zygomatic arch and body of zygoma. The origin of the zygomaticus major muscle is located at the main zygomatic retaining ligament. © Dr. Levent Efe, CMI.

Key Point

Injections superficial to the orbicularis muscle between the ORL and ZCL have the potential to disrupt the superficial lateral lymphatic chain of the midface leading to fluid collection between the cutaneous insertions of these ligaments. The end result is an iatrogenic malar mound.

3.5 Anterior Lower Midface

The zygomaticus major muscle acts as lateral boundary of the lower midface. The bony pyriform aperture serves as the medial boundary of the lower midface. The deep pyriform space (DPS) is a potential gliding space inferior to the lip elevator muscles and is the most medial deep injection target in the lower midface. The DPS is separated from the DMCF by the infraorbital neurovascular

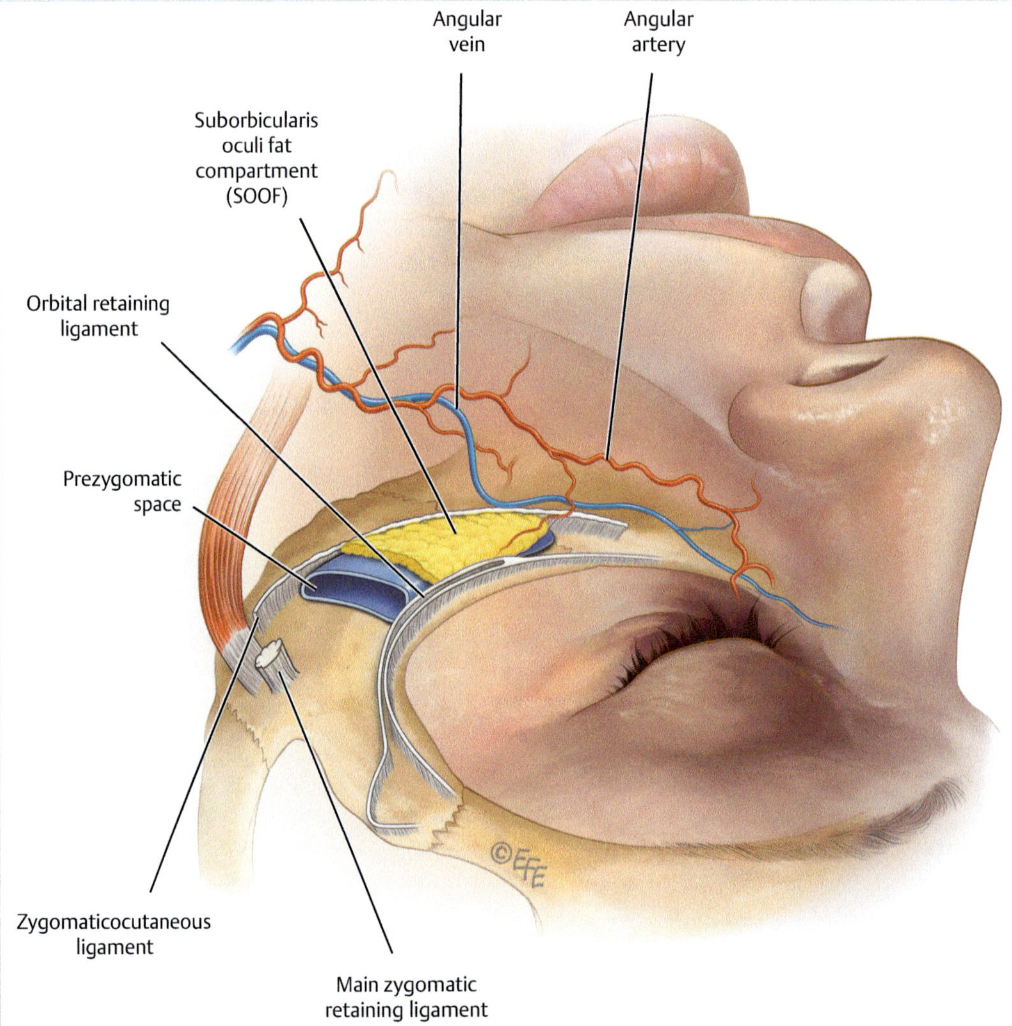

Fig. 3.5 Anatomic illustration of the angular artery residing medial to the orbital retaining ligament (ORL) and zygomaticocutaneous ligaments (ZCL) as well as the angular vein which travels through the buccal space and travels on the undersurface of the ZCL traversing medial to the tear trough ligament, eventually communicating with the dorsal nasal vein. The suborbicularis oculi fat (SOOF) is depicted. © Dr. Levent Efe, CMI.

bundle, which exits the maxilla through the superiorly hooded infraorbital foramen. The DMCF and DPS are well established targets for anterior cheek volumization. The DMCF is separated from the deep lateral cheek fat (DLCF) by the angular vein, which traverses from the facial vein canal in the buccal fat superiorly between the DMCF and DLCF continuing along the undersurface of the ZCL toward the tear trough. The DLCF and the buccal fat are divided by the zygomaticus major muscle (ZM).

Research has shown that the deep fat compartments of the face deflate with age leading to loss of soft tissue support and contour. Targeting these compartments during injection procedures can help to restore volume and shape that have been lost during the aging process. Note the superior labial nerve branch of the infraorbital nerve travels through the DPS so clinically injections in the DPS with anesthetic-infused filler products can lead to temporary numbness in the ipsilateral upper lip.

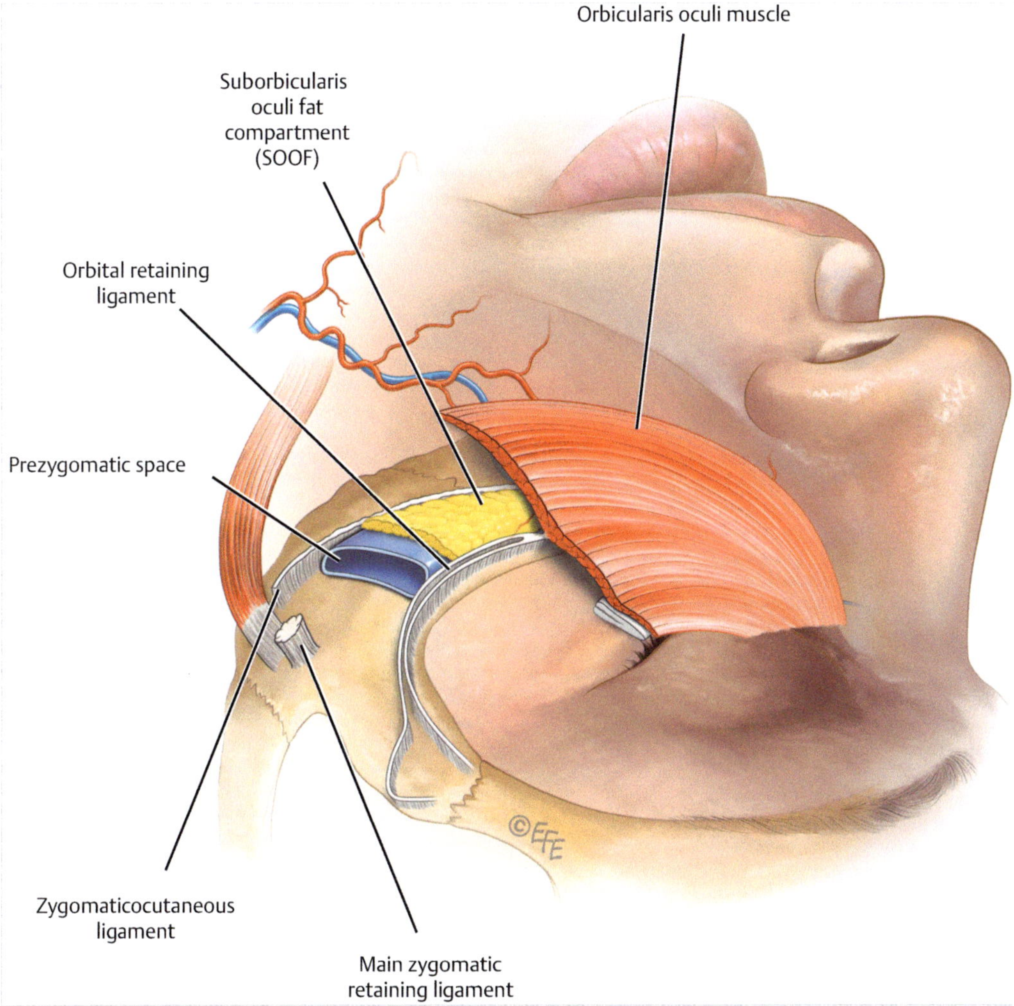

Fig. 3.6 Anatomic illustration of the orbicularis oculi muscle, which is synonymous with the superficial musculoaponeurotic system (SMAS) and forms the anterior/superficial boundary of the prezygomatic space and suborbicularis oculi fat (SOOF). © Dr. Levent Efe, CMI.

The angular artery terminates at the pyriform aperture in approximately 32 to 35% of cases. The angular artery is commonly located 3.3 cm lateral to nasal ala. Research has shown single branch angular arteries in 90% of cases, two branches in 9%, and three branches in 1% of cases. Angular arteries that continue into the alar facial groove often transition from the SMAS to subcutaneous plane superficial to the deep cheek fat and DPS. About 4% of angular arteries have been shown to travel deep to the SMAS near the periosteum of the maxilla. Caution should be taken when injecting anterior in the cheek, and pre-procedure vascular screening may be beneficial to assess for vascular variability in the pyriform region (▶ Fig. 3.9, ▶ Fig. 3.10, ▶ Fig. 3.11, ▶ Fig. 3.12).

3.6 The Tear Trough

The tear trough consists of three layers, namely, orbital rim bone, orbicularis oculi muscle, and skin. The tear tough ligament (TTL) is the medial

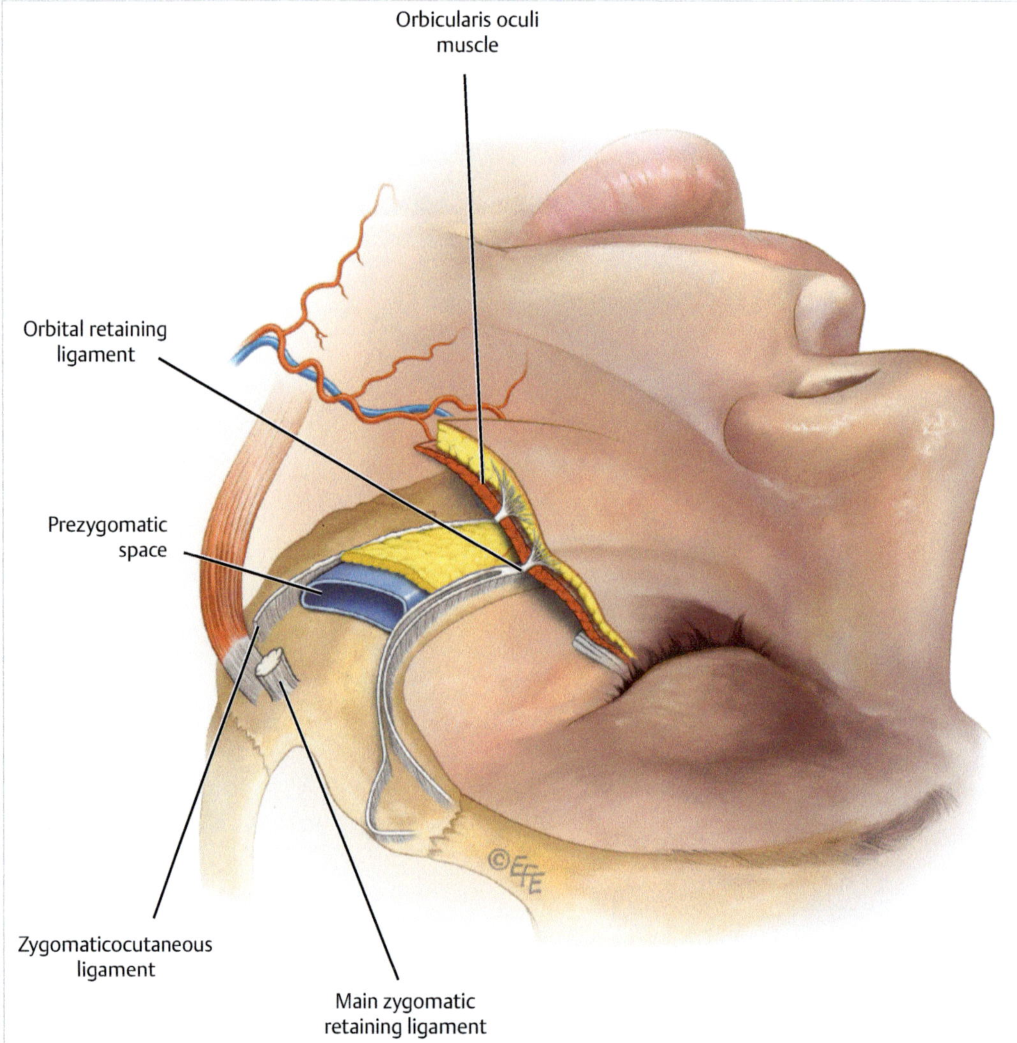

Fig. 3.7 Anatomic illustration of the cutaneous insertions of the zygomaticocutaneous ligaments and the orbicularis retaining ligament forming the surface topographic landmarks of the nasojugal groove and lid–cheek junction, respectively. © Dr. Levent Efe, CMI.

coalescence of the ORL and ZCL. The TTL travels from bone to skin and splits the orbital and palpebral leaflets of the orbicularis oculi. The angular vein and angular artery (if present) travel immediately medial to the TTL to anastomose with the dorsal nasal vasculature. Clinical injections that do not stay within the TTL can result in product deposition in the orbicularis oculi muscle, the lower eyelid preseptal space (superiorly), DPS (inferiorly), or in close proximity to the angular vessels (▶ Fig. 3.13, ▶ Fig. 3.14, ▶ Fig. 3.15, ▶ Fig. 3.16).

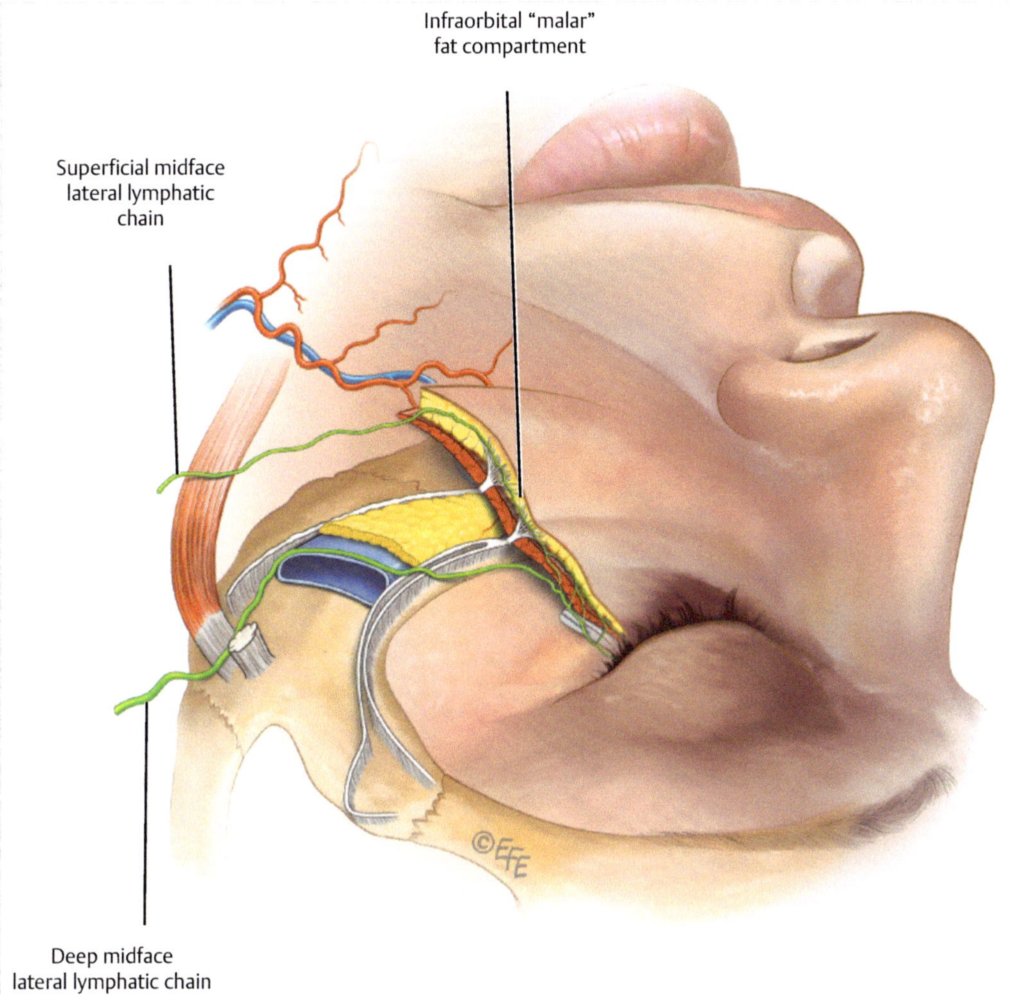

Fig. 3.8 Anatomic illustration of the midface lymphatic pathways. The lateral midface lymphatics contain a superficial chain that traverses through the malar fat compartment and a deep chain that drains through the floor of the prezygomatic space. © Dr. Levent Efe, CMI.

Key Point

Precision is key in clinical injections targeted at the tear trough ligament. Misplaced product may end up in the lower eyelid preseptal space, orbicularis oculi muscle, DPS, or in proximity of the angular artery and vein. The angular artery and vein anastomose with the dorsal nasal vessels, which contain direct connections to the ophthalmic vasculature.

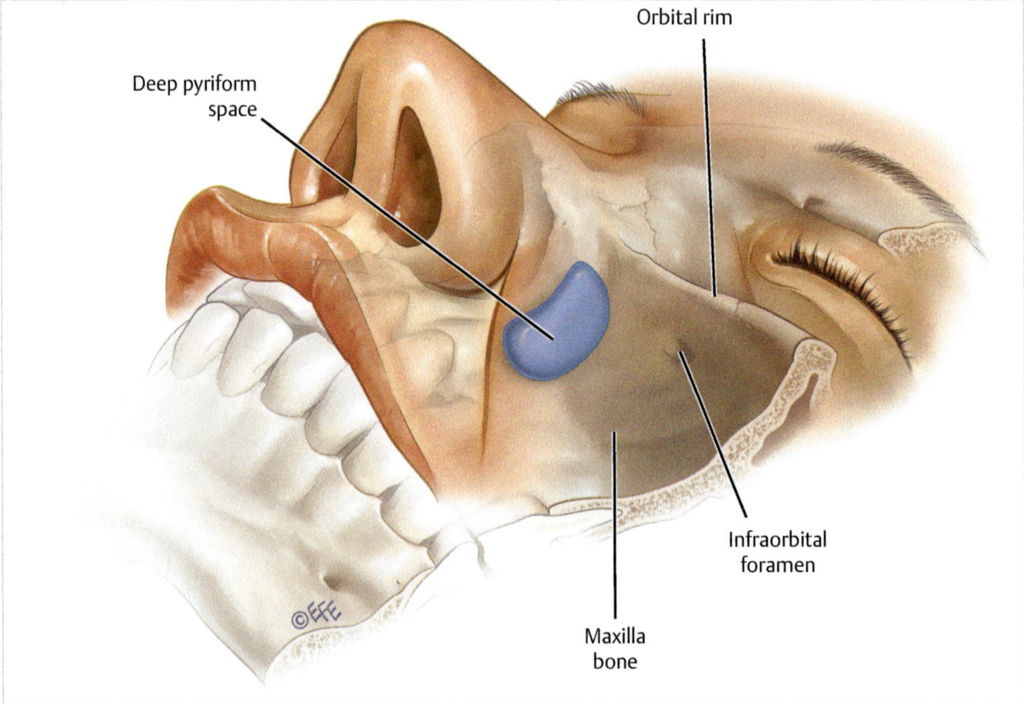

Fig. 3.9 Anatomic illustration of the anterior medial midface demonstrating the maxillary depression, deep pyriform space (DPS), and infraorbital foramen. © Dr. Levent Efe, CMI.

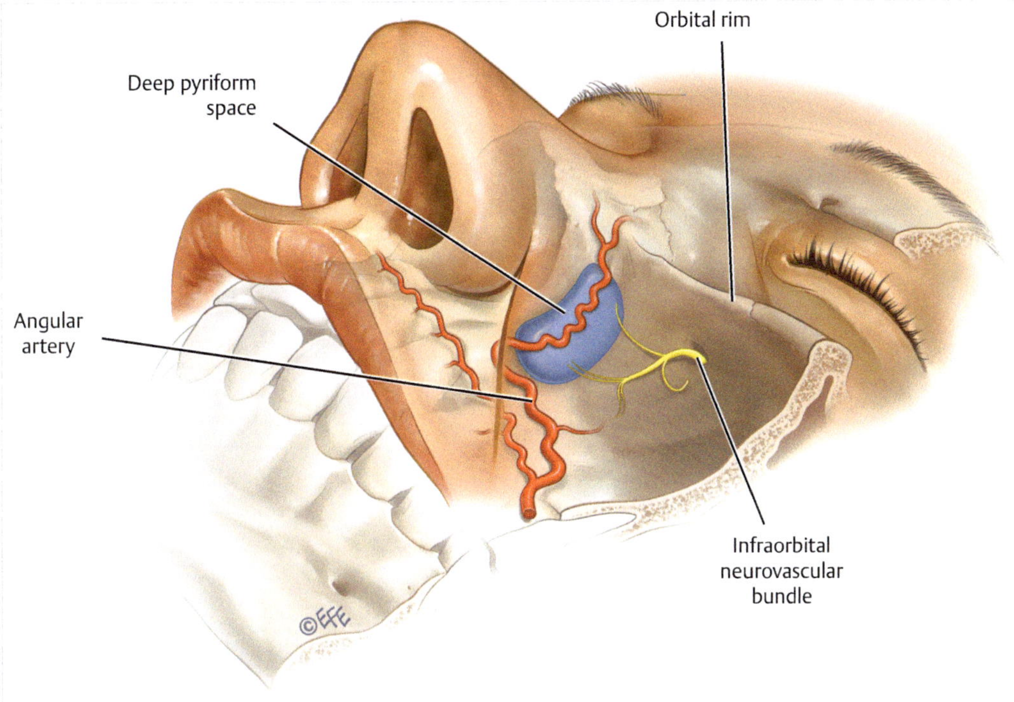

Fig. 3.10 Anatomic illustration of the anterior medial midface demonstrating the angular artery traversing across the medial third of the nasolabial fold and superficial to the deep pyriform space as well as the infraorbital nerve with four sensory branches, and the superior labial nerve branch traveling through the deep pyriform space and innervating the ipsilateral upper lip. © Dr. Levent Efe, CMI.

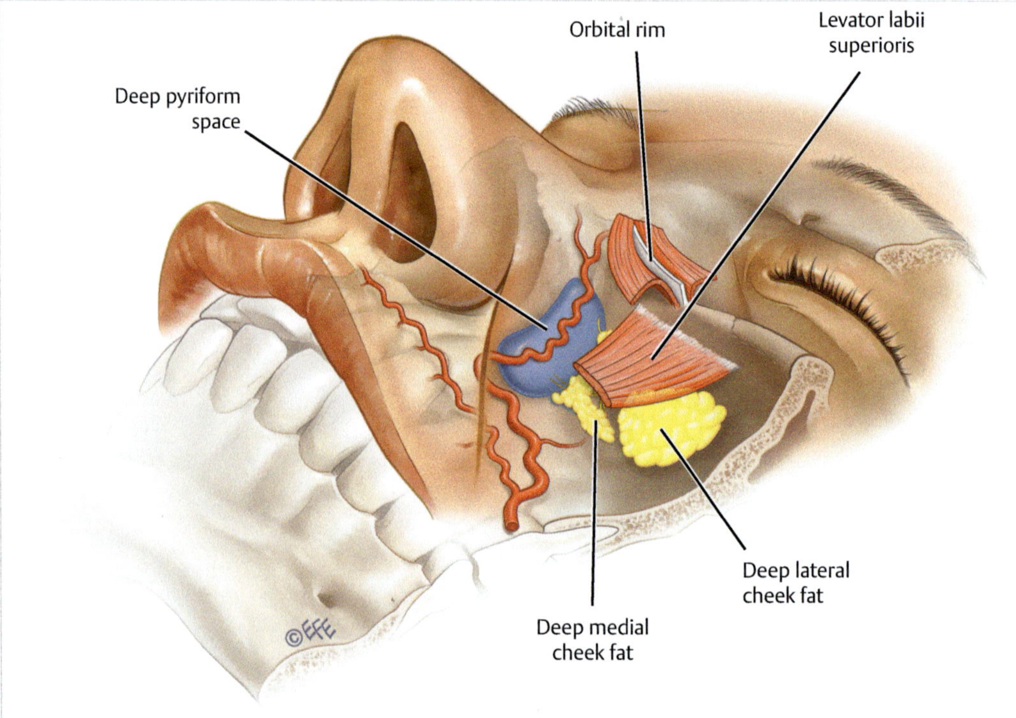

Fig. 3.11 Anatomic illustration of the anterior medial midface demonstrating the deep medial and deep lateral cheek fat as well as the levator labii superiorus which lies in the superficial musculoaponeurotic system (SMAS) layer superficial to the deep facial fat. © Dr. Levent Efe, CMI.

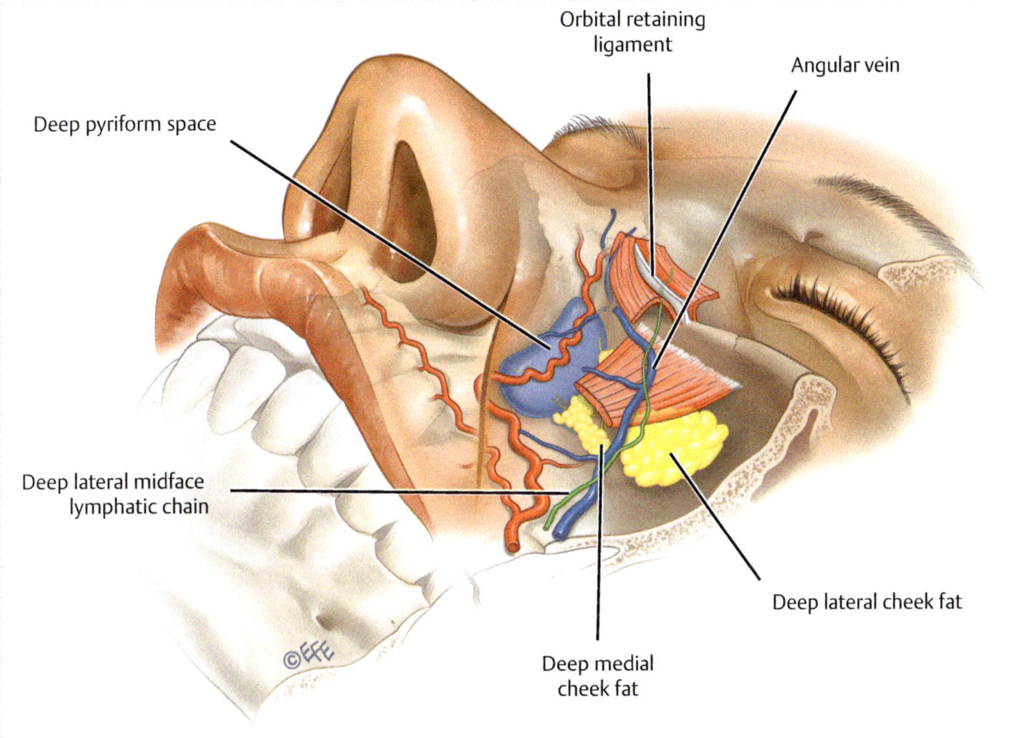

Fig. 3.12 Anatomic illustration of the anterior medial midface demonstrating the angular vein pathway through the buccal space and traveling on the undersurface of the zygomaticocutaneous ligaments and medial to the location where the orbital retaining ligament coalesces with the tear trough ligament. © Dr. Levent Efe, CMI.

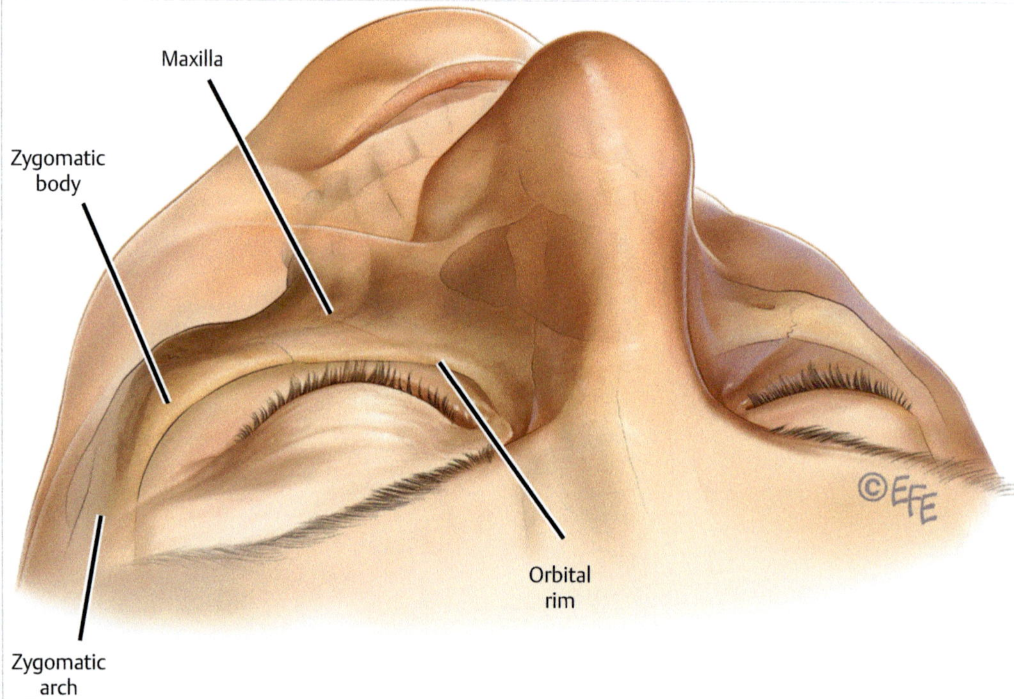

Fig. 3.13 Anatomic illustration of the tear trough region demonstrating the bony anatomy including the orbital rim, maxilla, body of zygoma, and zygomatic arch. © Dr. Levent Efe, CMI.

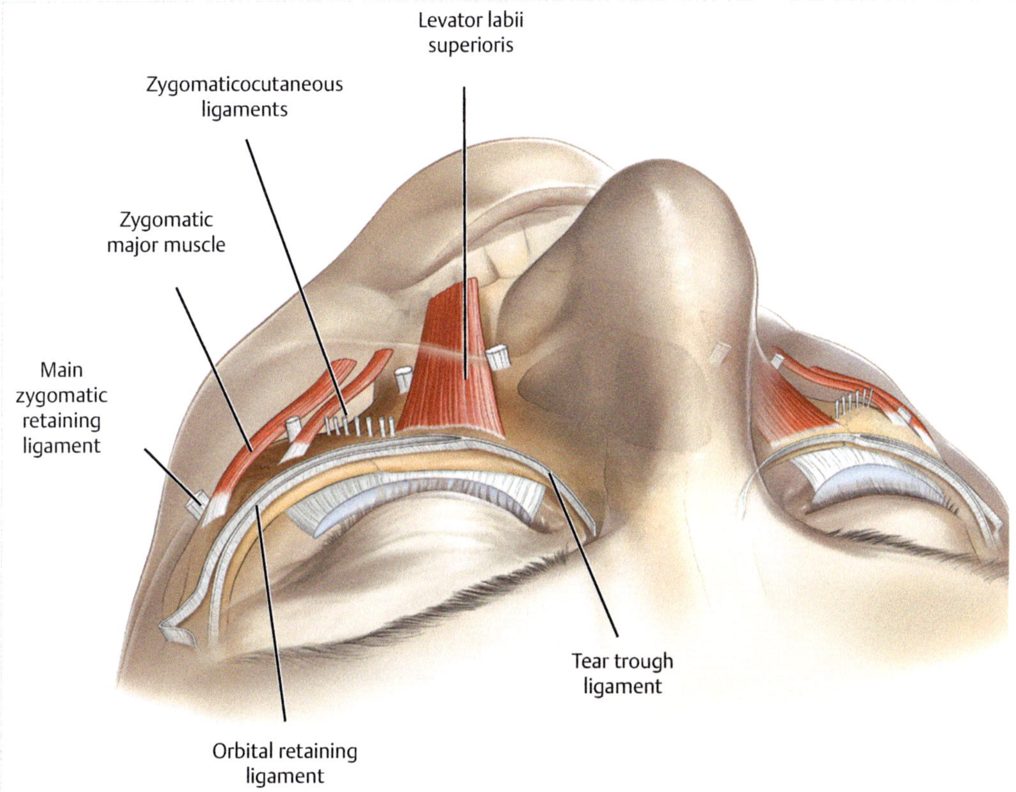

Fig. 3.14 Anatomic illustration of the tear trough region demonstrating the orbital retaining ligament and zygomaticocutenaous ligaments forming the tear trough ligament. Note the arcus marginalis which is the insertion of the orbital septum on the bony orbital rim and floor. © Dr. Levent Efe, CMI.

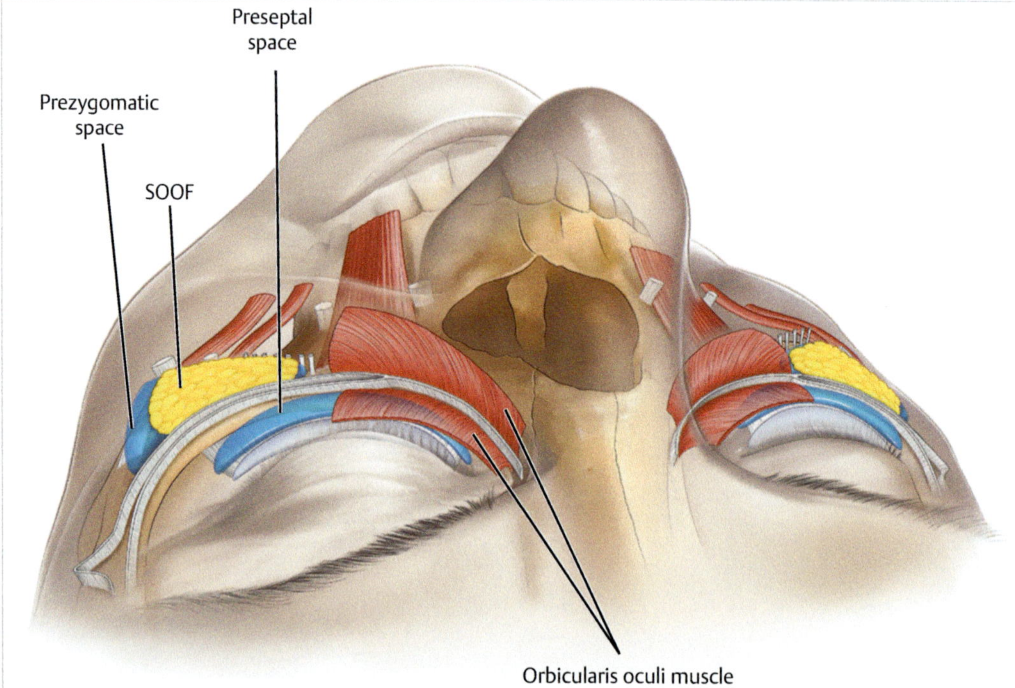

Fig. 3.15 Anatomic illustration of the tear trough region demonstrating the tear trough ligament splicing the orbital and palpebral leaflets of the orbicularis oculi muscle as well as the preseptal space of the lower eyelid residing above the orbital retaining ligament (ORL) and the prezygomatic space and suborbicularis oculi fat (SOOF) compartment residing between the ORL and zygoamticocutaneous ligaments (ZCL) respectively. © Dr. Levent Efe, CMI.

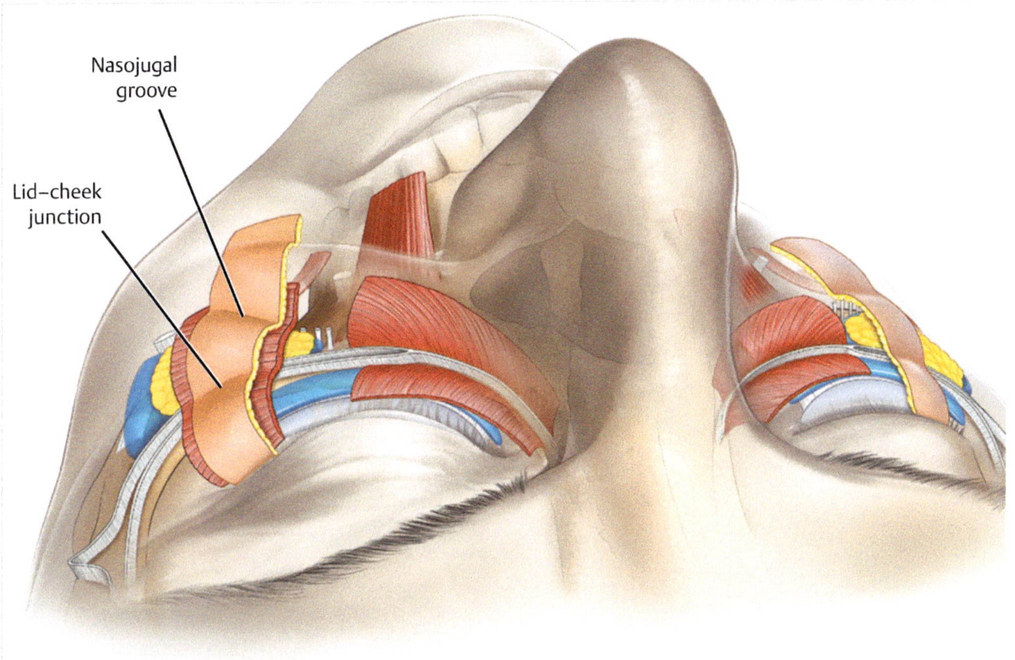

Fig. 3.16 Anatomic illustration of the tear trough region demonstrating the skin and associated surface topography. The cutaneous insertions of the zygomaticocutaneous ligaments (ZCL) form the nasojugal groove, and the cutaneous insertions of the orbital retaining ligament forms the lid–cheek junction and palpebromalar groove. © Dr. Levent Efe, CMI.

3.7 Ultrasound Anatomy and Technique for the Midface and Tear Trough

The most critical aspect for ultrasound imaging in the midface is determining the position and depth of the angular artery(s) in the DPS. The artery is a high-flow vessel so gain and scale can be in medium range or less. Although the current literature states the rate of a submuscular/supraperiosteal vessel is approximately 2 to 4%, in the author's (S.W.) experience, this is significantly low and may be closer to 30% or higher. Angular artery is absent in the DPS is approximately 30% of cases. In 9% of cases, there will be two branches and in 1% of cases, three branches. This is more common in females than in males. The injector must consider an alternate technique (other than needle directly on bone) if the angular artery lies along the periosteum such as ultrasound-guided injection or a more superficial placement of filler using needle or cannula.

One of the most pertinent structures to the injector is the SMAS, which is easily visualized using ultrasound as a hyperechoic linear structure at 3 to 5 mm depth. In the author's opinion, injections in the medial and lateral midface should generally be deep to the SMAS for safety, cosmetic result, and longevity of the filler. The prezygomatic space can be visualized using ultrasound and is the ideal location for midface injections. Medial to the space is the angular vein and artery, and inferiorly is the infraorbital foramen with its infraorbital artery, vein, and nerve.

Tear trough ultrasound demonstrates the very tight space in which an injector is required to place filler and underscores the high rate of removal of filler due to improper placement and/or spread of the filler (▶ Fig. 3.17, ▶ Fig. 3.18, ▶ Fig. 3.19, ▶ Fig. 3.20, ▶ Fig. 3.21, ▶ Fig. 3.22, ▶ Fig. 3.23, ▶ Fig. 3.24, ▶ Fig. 3.25, ▶ Fig. 3.26, ▶ Fig. 3.27, ▶ Fig. 3.28, ▶ Fig. 3.29, ▶ Fig. 3.30, ▶ Fig. 3.31, ▶ Fig. 3.32, ▶ Fig. 3.33, ▶ Fig. 3.34, ▶ Fig. 3.35, ▶ Fig. 3.36, ▶ Fig. 3.37, ▶ Fig. 3.38, ▶ Fig. 3.39, ▶ Fig. 3.40, ▶ Fig. 3.41, ▶ Fig. 3.42).

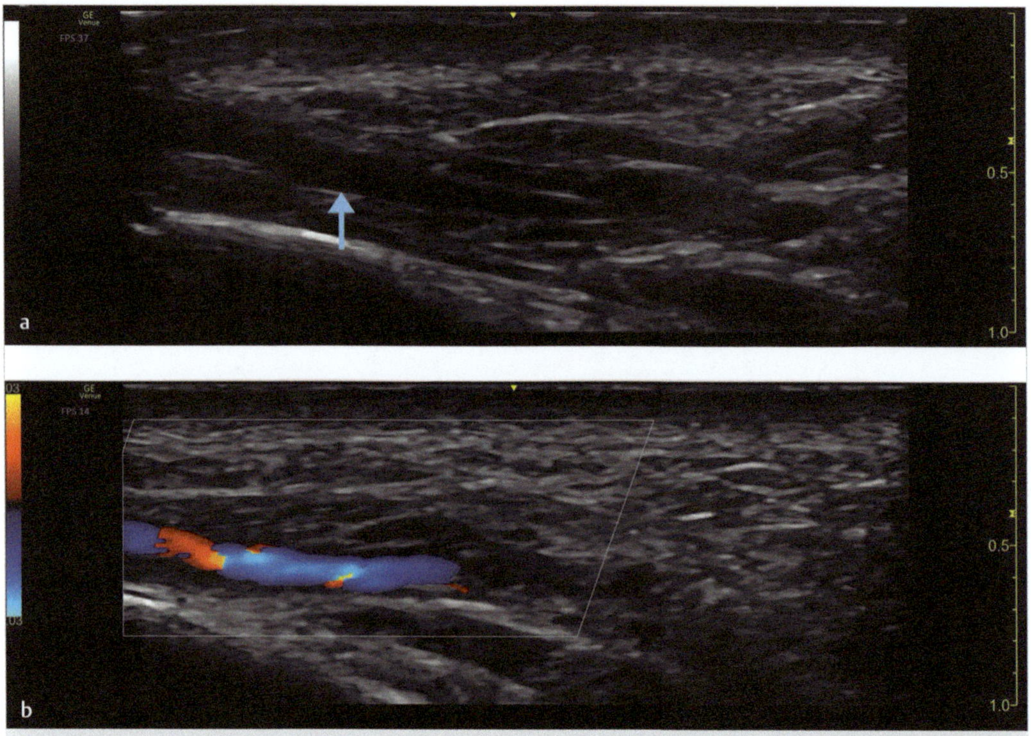

Fig. 3.17 **(a, b)** Images obtained with an 18-MHz probe in vertical position. This is the angular vein (blue arrow) in the medial canthal area. It lies medial to the tear trough ligament. This can often be much larger than the angular artery and is valveless, creating a pathway into the cavernous sinus or ophthalmic system. Upper image is B mode. The angular vein is found lateral to angular artery in the medial canthal area.

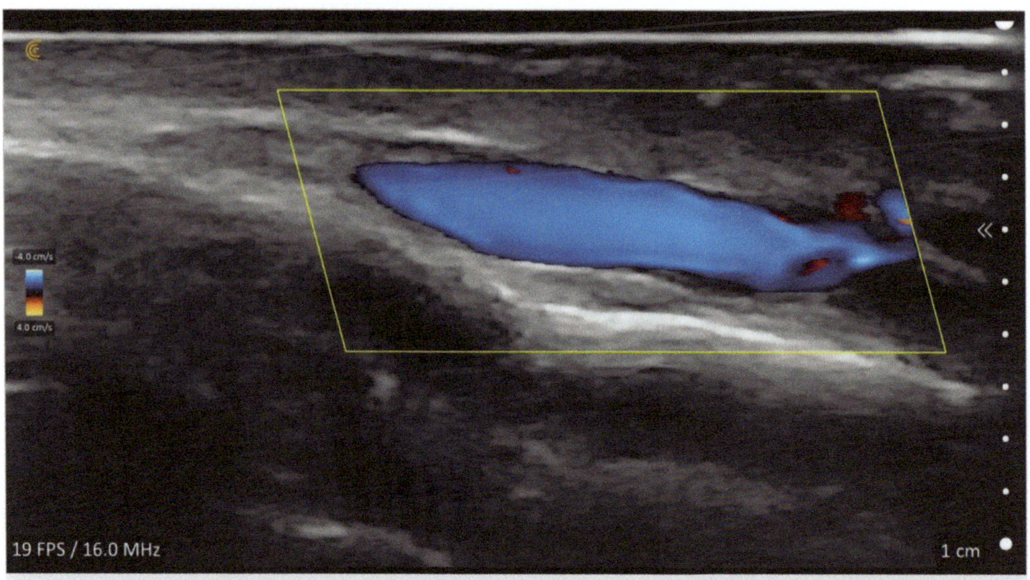

Fig. 3.18 Image obtained using a 20-MHz handheld probe in vertical position using color Doppler. Note large angular vein in medial canthal area.

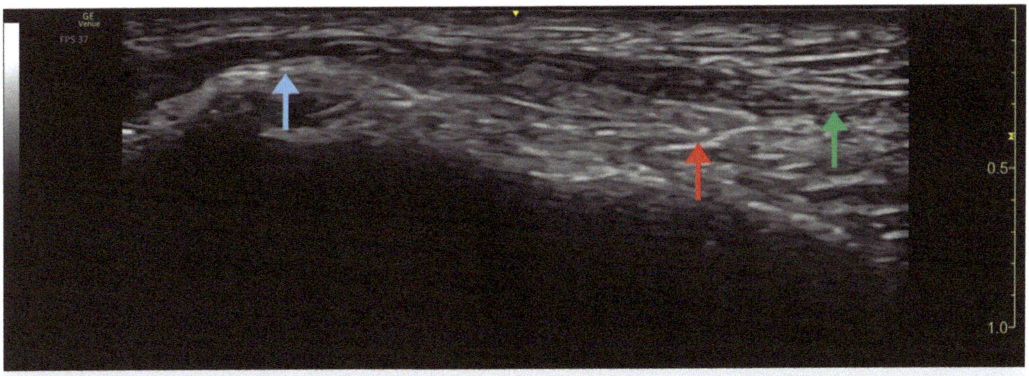

Fig. 3.19 Image obtained using an 18-MHz horizontal probe. The tear trough area is shown (blue arrow). Note that in this area, there is bone, muscle, and skin only. The medial suborbicularis oculi fat (SOOF) pad is shown (red arrow) below the hypoechoic orbicularis oculi (green arrow).

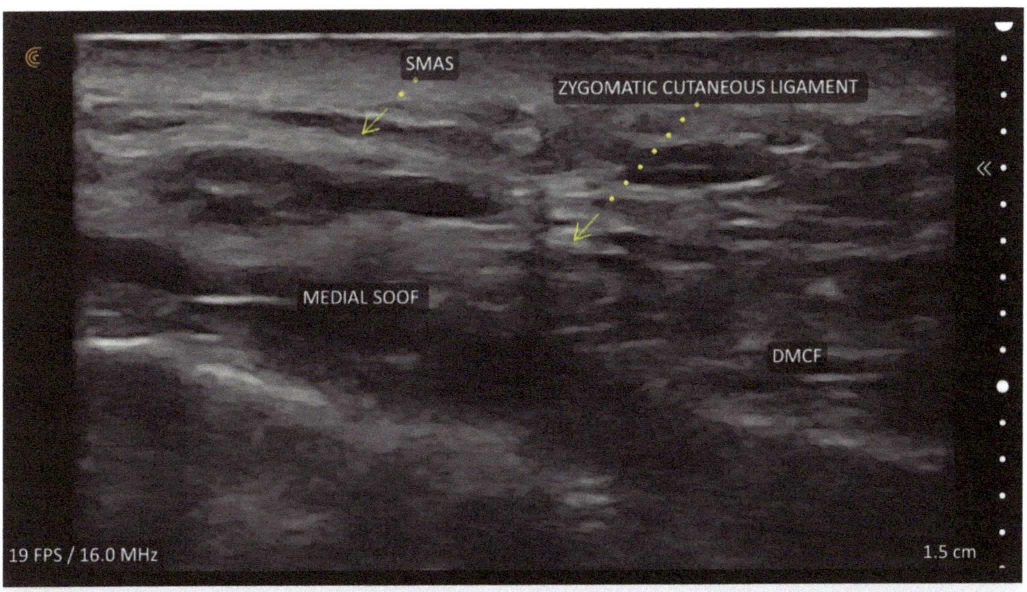

Fig. 3.20 Image obtained using a 20-MHz handheld vertical probe, superior to the left. The zygomaticocutaneous (ZC) ligament runs from the periosteum to the skin and is hyperechoic due to its collagen component. Superior to the ZC ligament is the medial suborbicularis oculi fat (SOOF) pad and inferior is the deep medial cheek fat (DMCF). Superficial to these fat pads is the superficial musculoaponeurotic system (SMAS), which is contiguous with the orbicularis oculi in the superior cheek. Superficial to the SMAS is the superficial fat pad. It is often more echogenic than the deep fat pad because of the higher content of fibrous tissue.

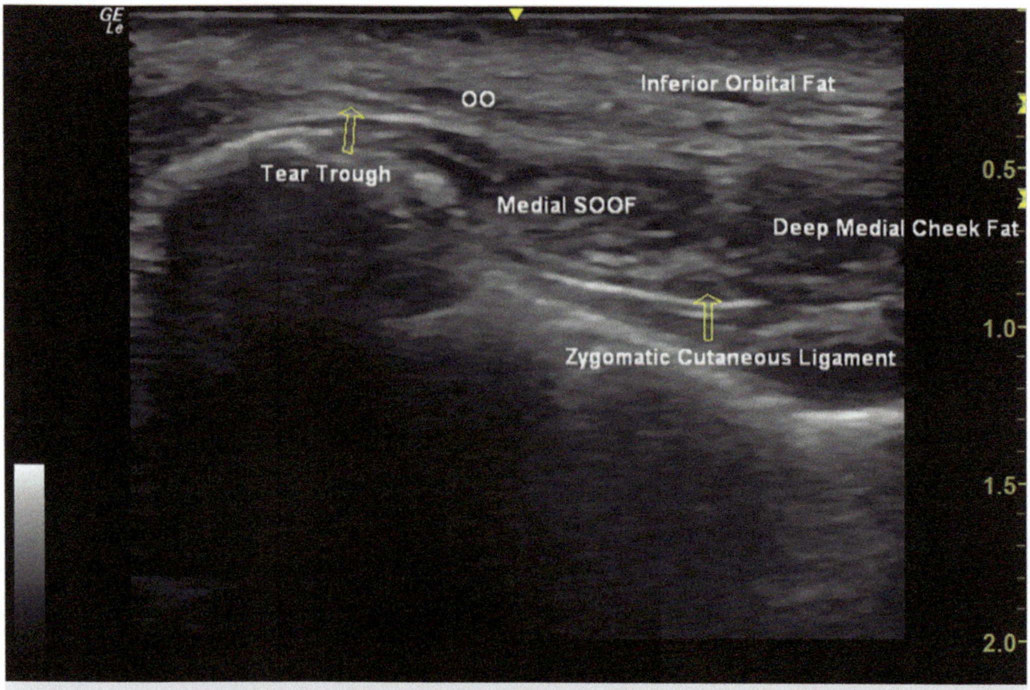

Fig. 3.21 Image obtained using an 18-MHz vertical probe. This image is more medial than prior image showing zygomaticocutaneous ligament (ZC ligament) extending from the bone to skin and the medial suborbicularis oculi fat (SOOF) superior to the ligament and deep medial cheek fat lying inferior to the ligament. Note the malar fat pad (labeled inferior orbital fat) is more echogenic than the deep fat pads.

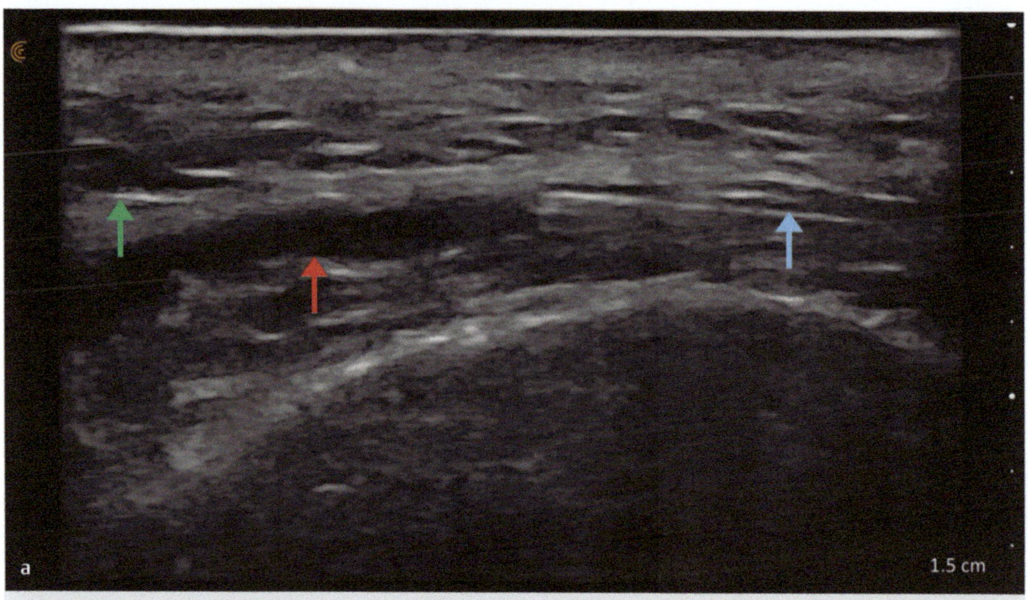

Fig. 3.22 **(a)** Image obtained using a 20-MHz handheld probe. Hyaluronic acid (HA) filler (red arrow) is placed with cannula (blue arrow) along the undersurface of the superficial musculoaponeurotic system (SMAS) (green arrow), in the prezygomatic space. The fat in the prezygomatic space is the medial suborbicularis oculi fat (SOOF). Superficial to the SMAS is the malar fat pad.

(Continued)

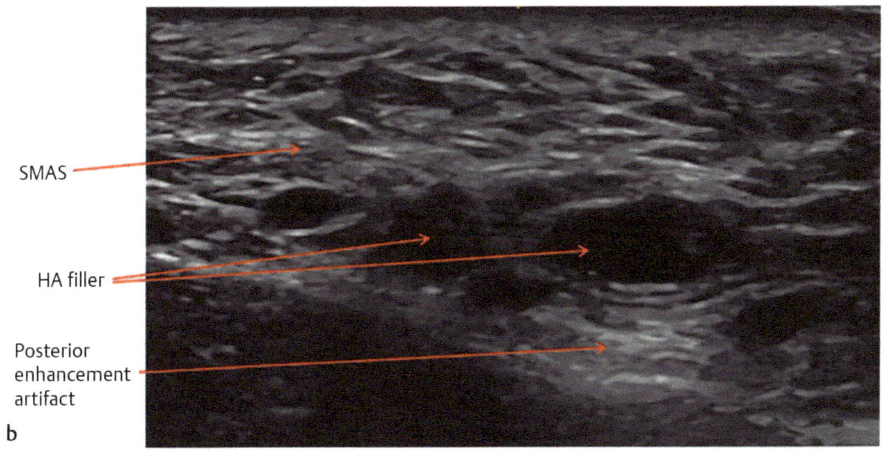

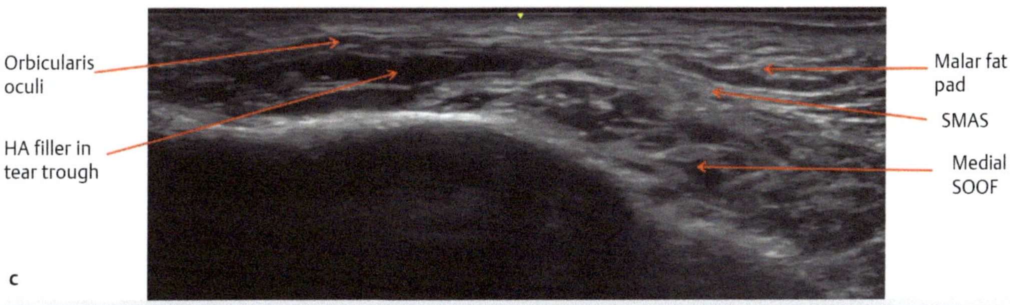

Fig. 3.22 (*Continued*) **(b)** Image obtained using a 20-MHz probe in a horizontal orientation in mid-cheek. HA filler after placement in the prezygomatic space with cannula. It is below the SMAS. Note that there is posterior enhancement artifact which is typical of HA filler. **(c)** Image obtain using a 20-MHz probe along the nasojugal groove (45 degree angle from mid cheek to tear trough). Note the filler is place beneath the orbicularis oculi in the tear trough (via cannula). Staying below the SMAS/Orbicularis oculi is important to minimize malar edema related to the filler (SW and CS opinion). Filler placed in the malar fat pad is associated with later complications such as malar and lower lid edema.

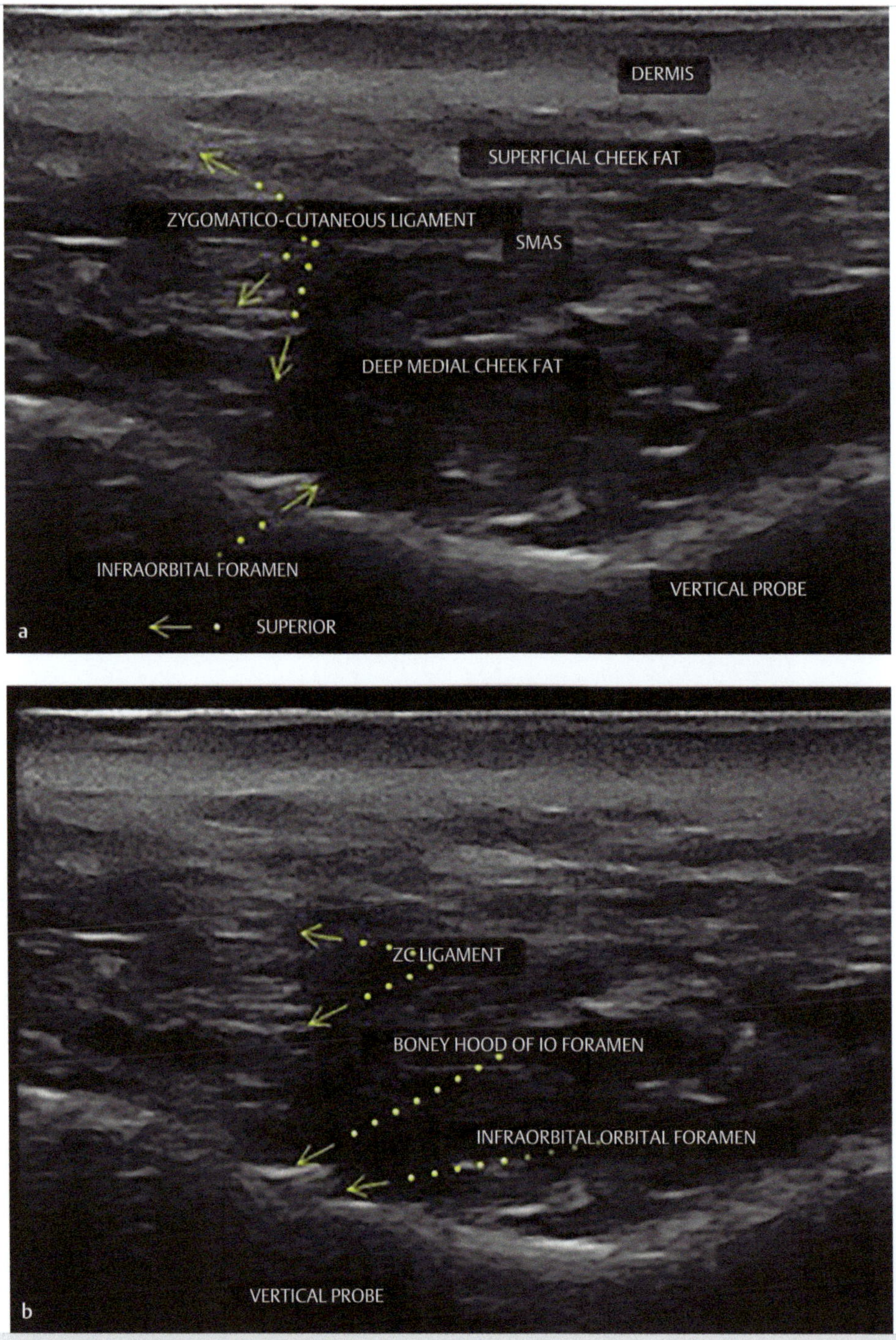

Fig. 3.23 (**a, b**) These images were obtained with a vertical 20-MHz probe in medial cheek near mid-pupillary line. Note the zygomatico-cutaneous ligament can be seen arising superior to the infraorbital foramen. The infraorbital foramen and artery are protected when injections are placed in the prezygomatic space by the ZC ligament. Also note the superior hood/lip of the infraorbital foramen which additionally protects the nerve and artery from inadvertent injury when injecting from a superior approach in the anterior cheek. There is an accessory foramen in 9% and 3 foramen in 0.5% of patients.

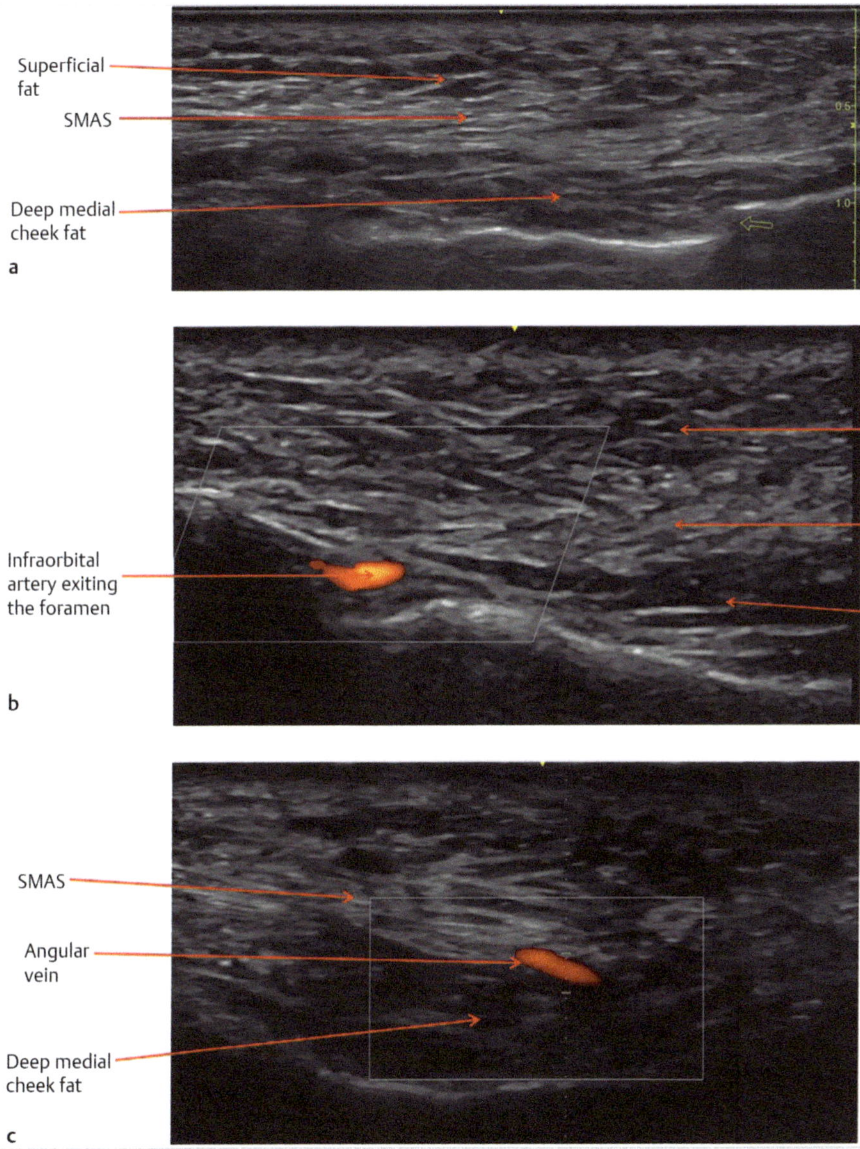

Fig. 3.24 (a, b) The first image above was obtained with a 20-MHz probe in a horizontal orientation on the mid anterior cheek and the next two were in a vertical orientation. The layers of the cheek can be seen in the first image with the yellow arrow pointing to the infraorbital foramen. The second image shows the infraorbital artery exiting the foramen and entering the deep medial cheek fat. The infraorbital artery is one of the deeper arteries in the face and often requires lower frequency probes (>12 MHz) for best visualization. Note that there is more fibrous tissue in the superficial fat which makes it more echogenic than the deep fat. **(c)** Image obtained using a 20-MHz probe in vertical position in mid anterior cheek using power doppler. Note that the angular vein (compressible) lies in a plane more superficial to the infraorbital artery. Also note that spectral doppler was used to determine this was a vein. In the mid-cheek, the angular vein is usually seen in close association with the SMAS layer. It can be distinguished from the artery because it is usually larger, more superficial, compressible, and has venous characteristics on spectral doppler analysis.

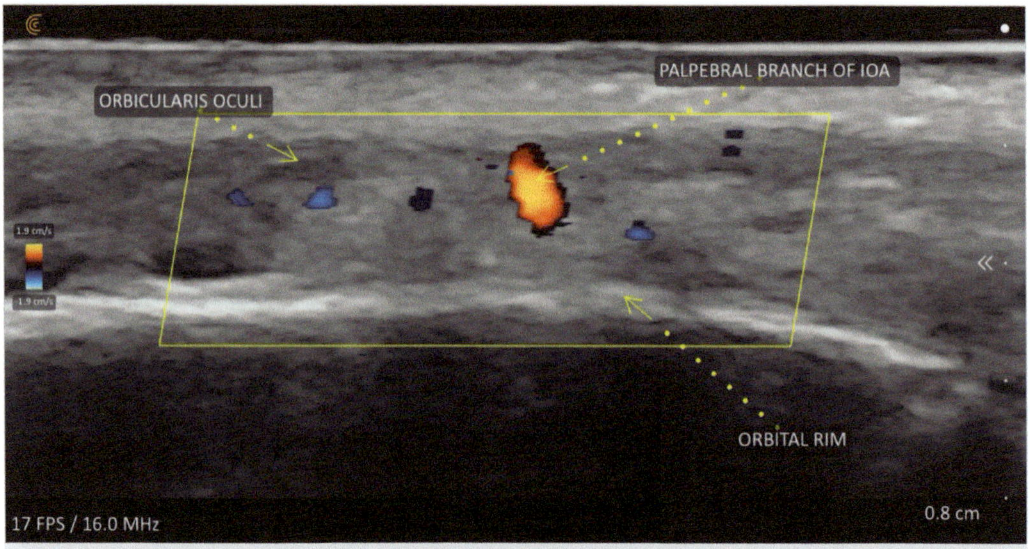

Fig. 3.25 Image obtained using a 20-MHz probe in horizontal position on the lower eyelid. The palpepral branch of the infraorbital artery (PIOA) is visualized, which runs superiorly from the infraorbital foramen and travels in the midpupillary line in the superficial fat to reach the lower eyelid. In needle injections onto the periosteum, care must be taken to avoid this artery, and it is recommended to inject medial to midpupillary line when injecting the tear trough.

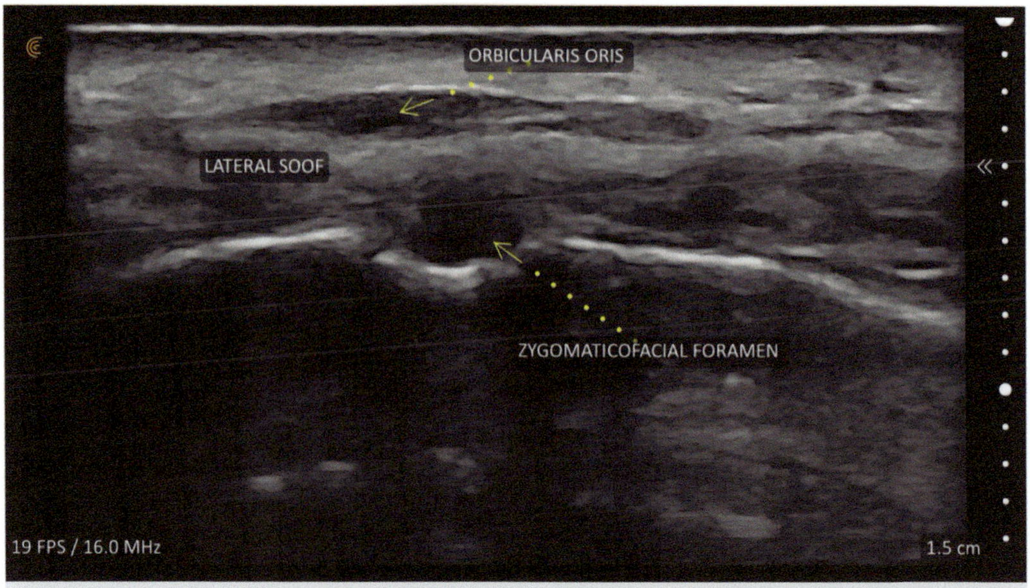

Fig. 3.26 Image obtained using a 20-MHz handheld probe in horizontal position. The zygomaticofacial foramen lies near the orbital rim on the lateral cheek. Overlying the foramen is the lateral suborbicularis oculi fat (SOOF), which is just deep to the orbicularis oculi muscle. There is a small superficial fat pad overlying the orbicularis oculi muscle and deep to dermis.

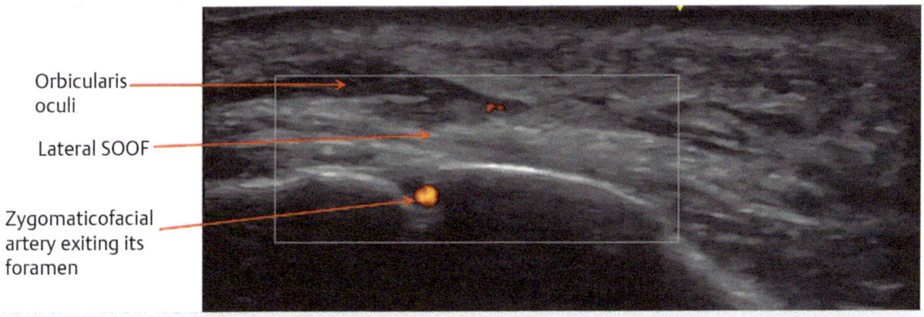

Fig. 3.27 Image obtained using an 20-MHz probe in horizontal position and power doppler. Visualization of the zygomaticofacial artery is often difficult due to its small size and low flow. This artery directly communicates with the eye and should be considered when injecting on the upper zygoma on periosteum. The discontinuity in the bone is how foramina are identified. OO, orbicularis oculi; SOOF, suborbicularis oculi fat.

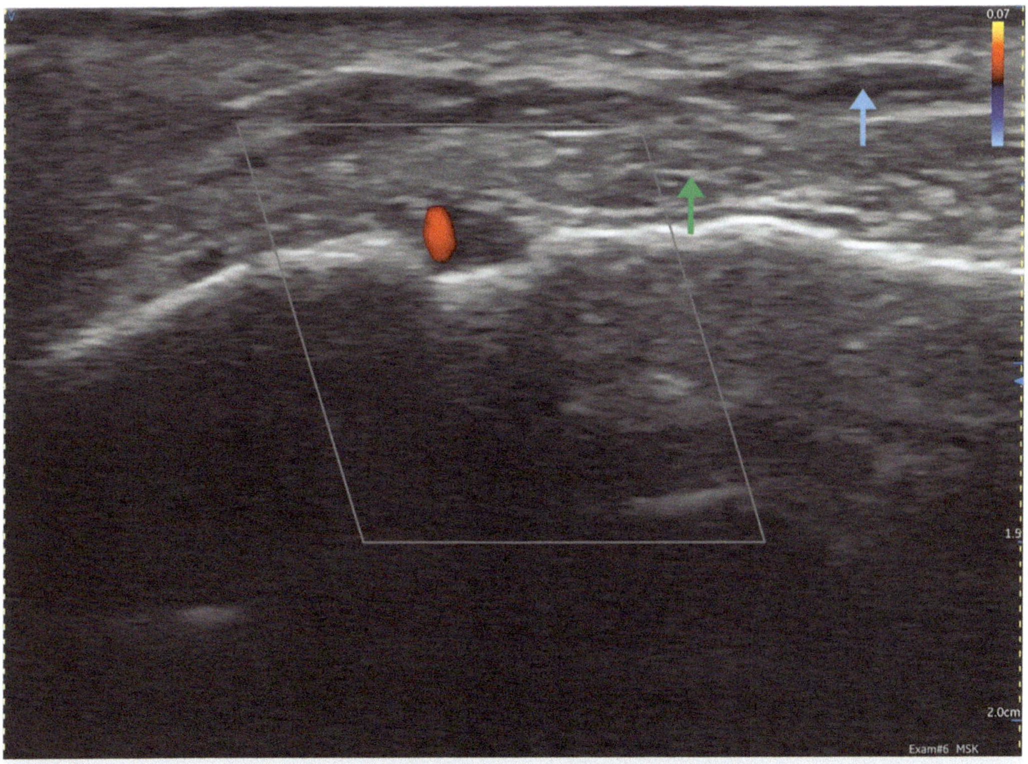

Fig. 3.28 Image obtained using a 12-MHz handheld probe. The zygomaticofacial artery is shown exiting the zygomaticofacial foramen. Orbicularis oculi muscle (blue arrow) and lateral suborbicularis oculi fat (SOOF) (green arrow) are shown as well. Low-flow vessels can sometimes be easier to visualize with a lower frequency probe.

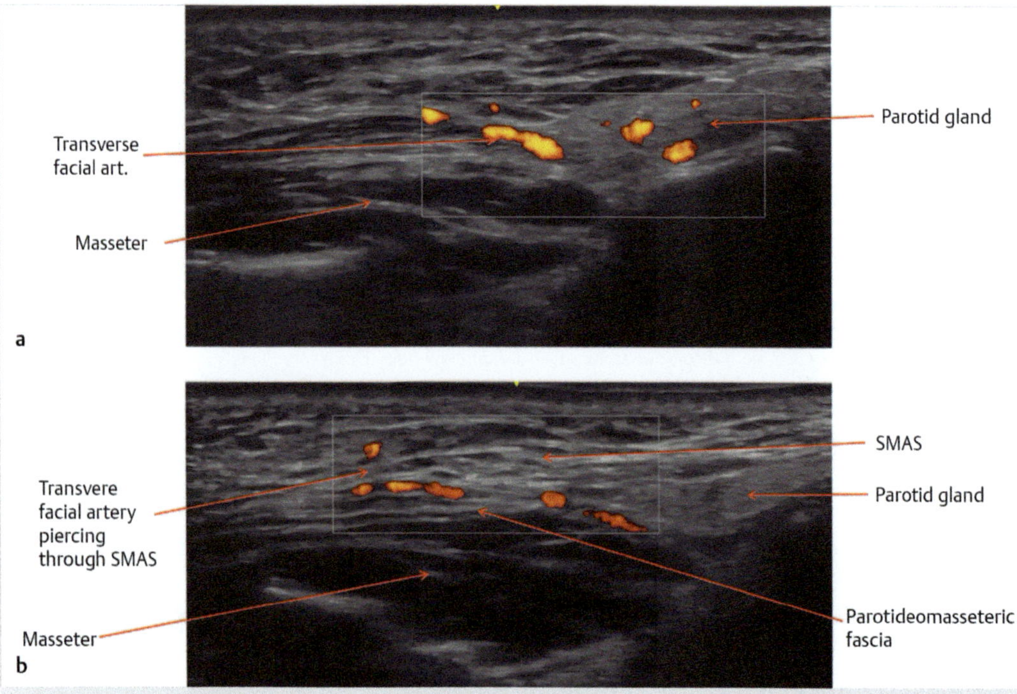

Fig. 3.29 (a, b) Images obtained using a 20-MHz probe in horizontal position using power doppler in the submalar area. The transverse facial artery is shown passing through the parotid gland. It can be a single or double vessel. It then travels medially along the parotideomasseteric fascia. Eventually, the artery pierces the superficial musculoaponeurotic system (SMAS) and travels in the superficial fat pad.

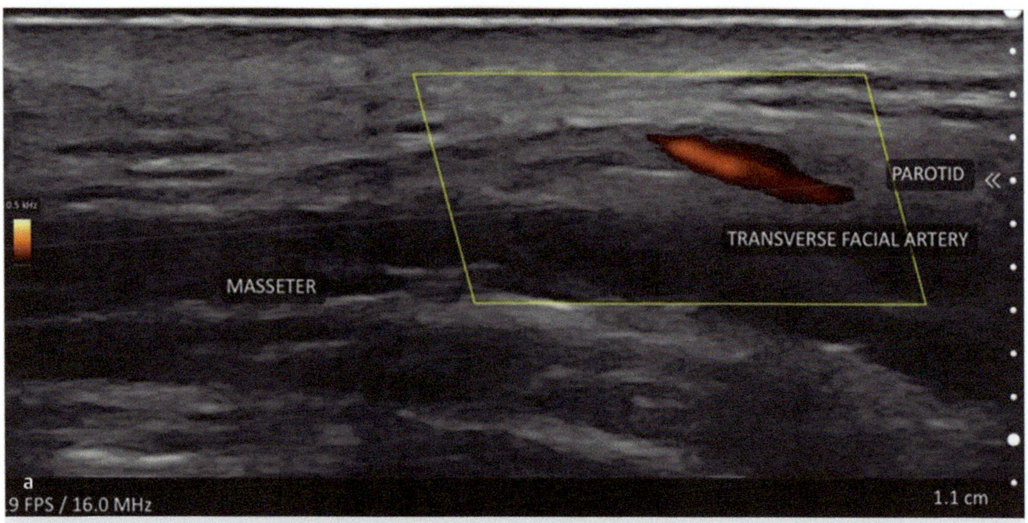

Fig. 3.30 (a, b) Image obtained using a 20-MHz handheld probe in power Doppler mode in a horizontal orientation in submalar region. Note isoechoic appearance of the parotid gland that is lying on the masseter. Lower image shows the two artery variant.

(Continued)

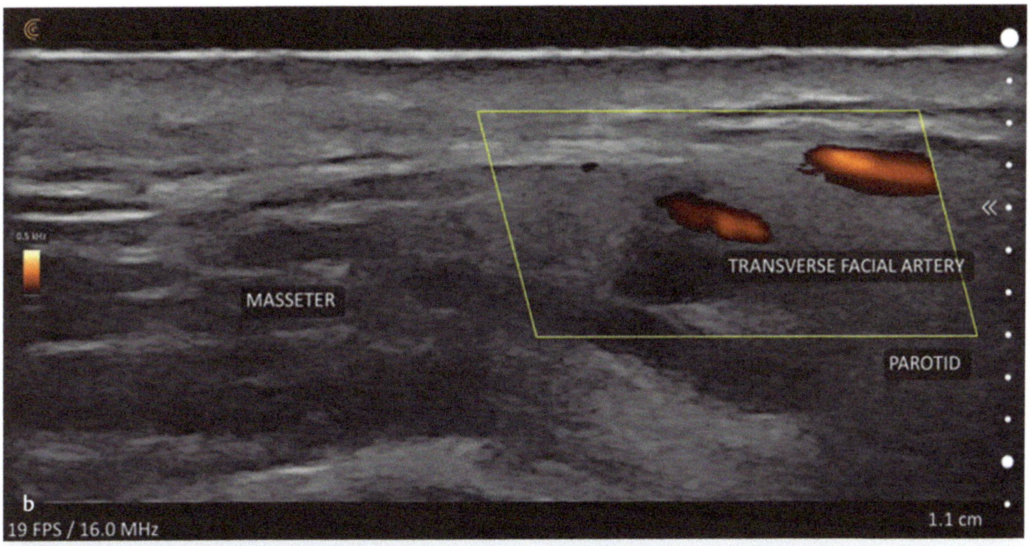

Fig. 3.30 (*Continued*) (**b**)

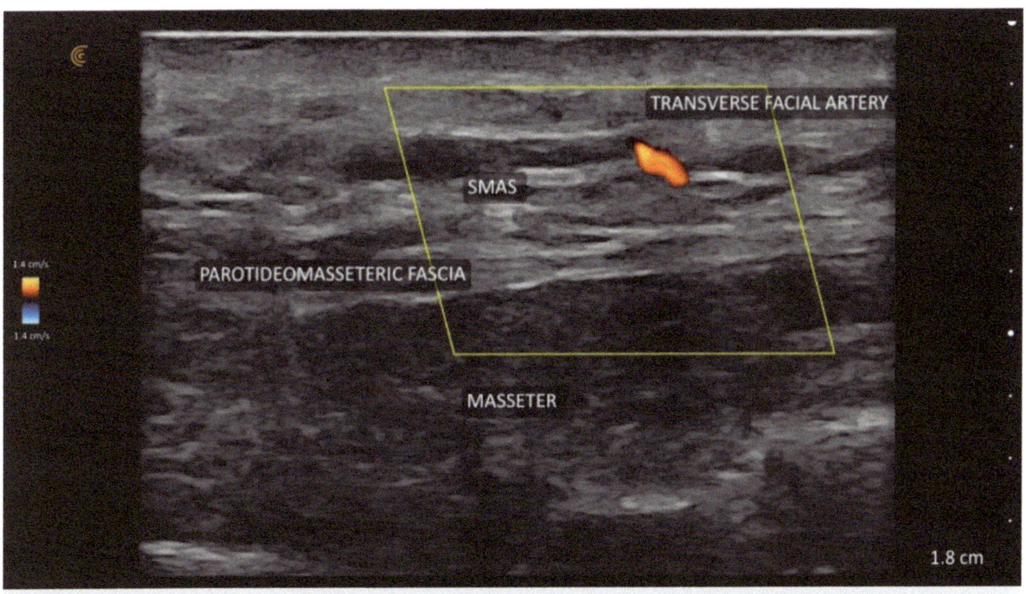

Fig. 3.31 Image obtained using a 20-MHz probe in a horizontal position. This image shows the transverse facial artery piercing the superficial musculoaponeurotic system (SMAS) to become more superficial in its position.

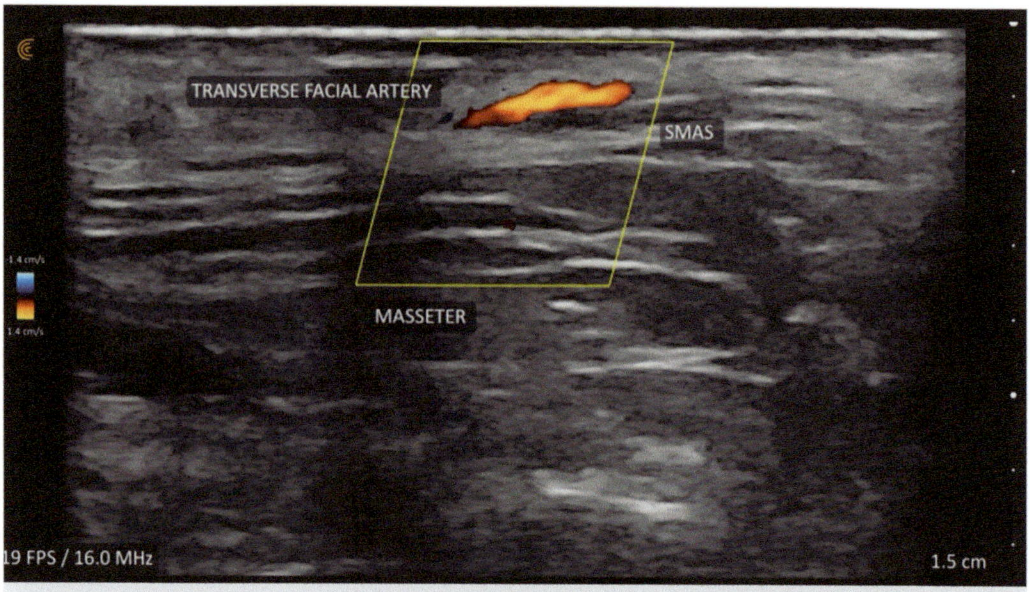

Fig. 3.32 Image obtained using a 20-MHz probe in horizontal position. This image shows the superficial aspect of the transverse facial artery in the subcutaneous fat, superficial to the superficial musculoaponeurotic system (SMAS) in the submalar area.

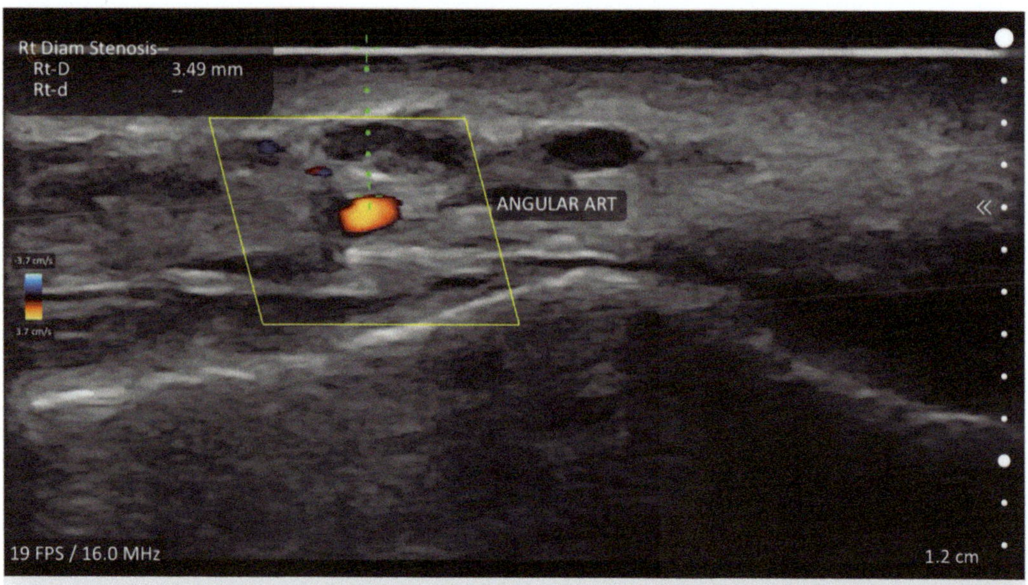

Fig. 3.33 This image is obtained with a 20-MHz handheld probe in 45 degrees angle resting on the lateral nasal ala. The angular artery is shown in the area of the deep pyriform space. It is typically 4 to 5 mm deep in this area. Ultrasound is critical to evaluate whether there is a supraperiosteal variant, which is reported in approximately 2% of cases in the literature.

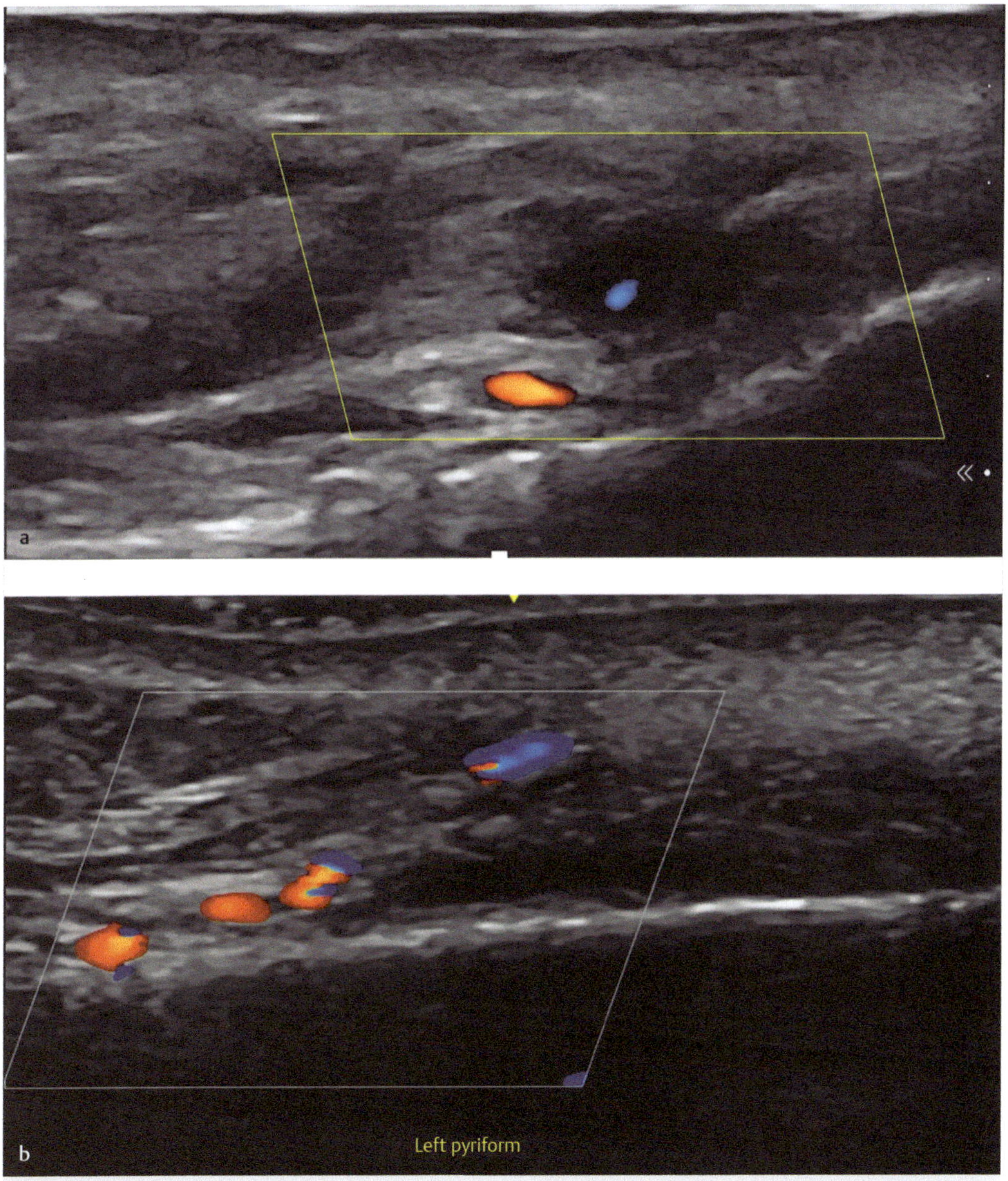

Fig. 3.34 **(a)** Similar settings to the image in ▶ Fig. 3.33. This image shows an angular artery variant with two branches in the deep pyriform area. This occurs in 9% of individuals. In the author's experience, if there are two (or three) branches, usually at least one is supraperiosteal. **(b)** Image obtained using a 20-MHz probe in oblique orientation next to alar rim. There are two angular arteries in the deep pyriform space with one branch along the periosteum and one in the SMAS layer.

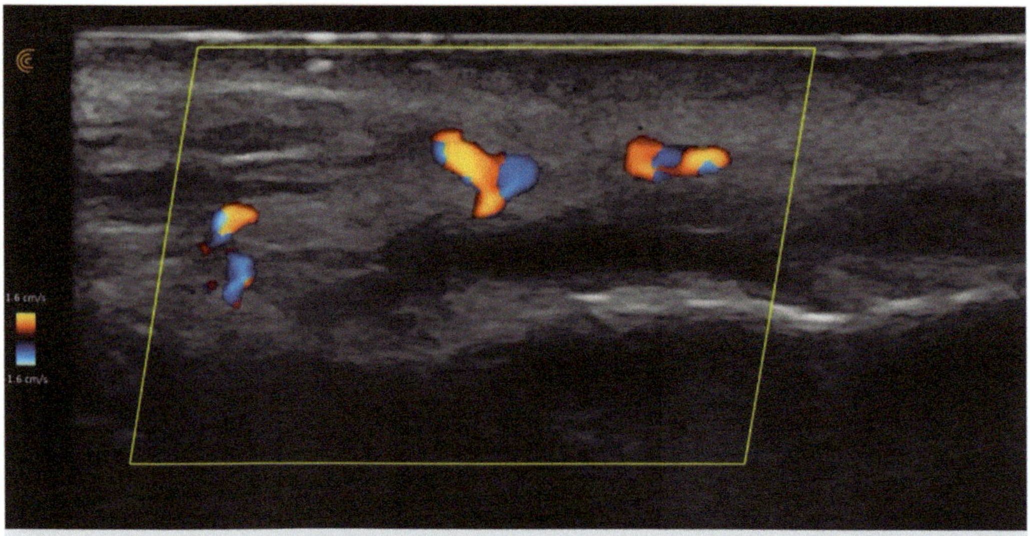

Fig. 3.35 Similar settings to the image in ▶ Fig. 3.33. This image shows the three-branch variant of the angular artery. This variant occurs approximately 1% of the time, and females tend to have the tendency to have multiple branches compared with males.

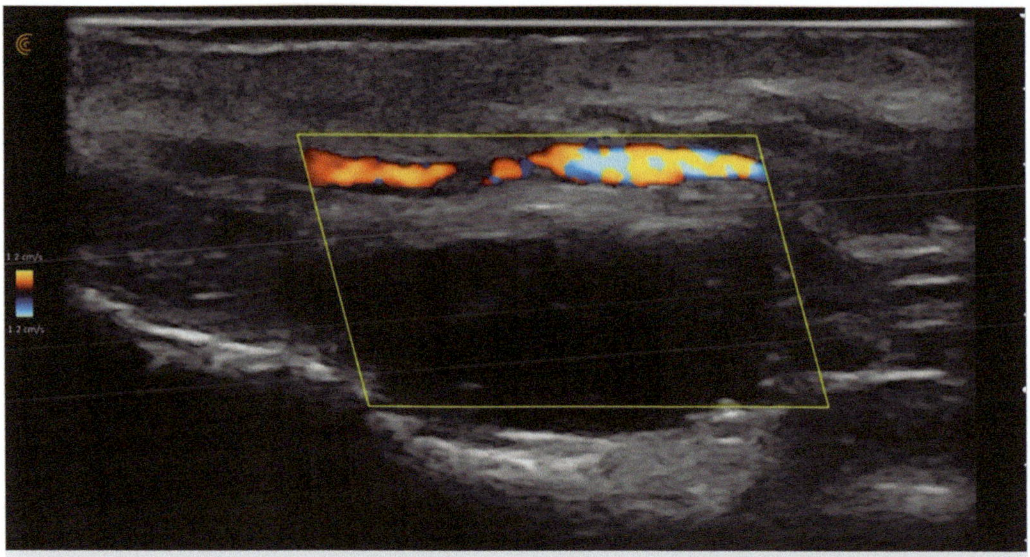

Fig. 3.36 Similar settings to the image in ▶ Fig. 3.33. The angular artery is seen resting on a hyaluronic acid filler bolus placed in the deep pyriform space. The bolus is placed directly on the periosteum using a needle.

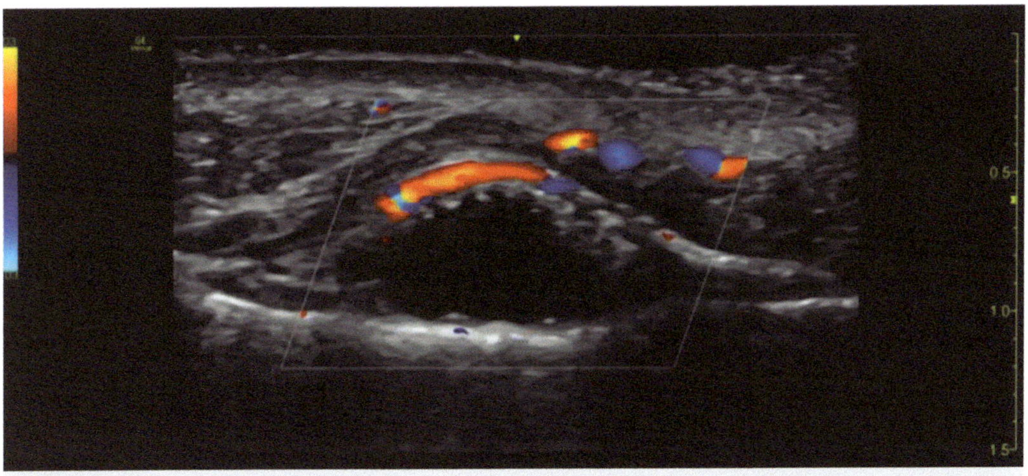

Fig. 3.37 Image obtained using an 18-MHz probe at 45 degrees against alar base. The angular artery is displaced by hyaluronic acid (HA) filler placed on periosteum with needle injection. Multiple branches of angular artery are present in this individual.

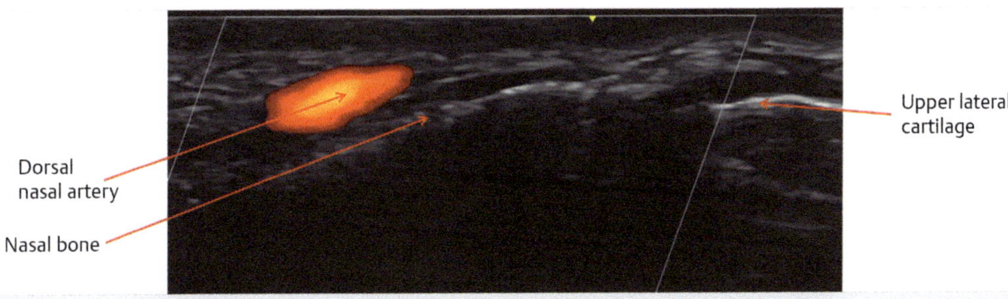

Fig. 3.38 Image obtained using a 18-MHz probe in a paramedian position oriented vertically on the nasal dorsum. The dorsal nasal artery will typically run in a paramedian position within the SMAS of the nose. In this image, the artery is not lying on the periosteum but very close. Even if the injector is placing their needle on the bone, the bevel might still lay within the vessel and not below it. In a paper by Alfershofer, Frank, Cotofana et al., the dorsal nasal artery was on the periosteum in 16.7% in the mid nasal dorsum and 1.7% in the nasal radix.

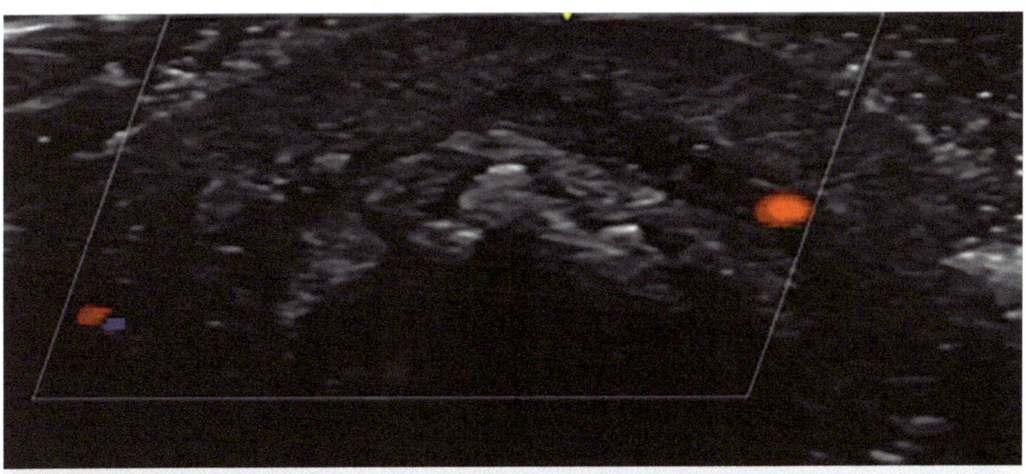

Fig. 3.39 Image obtained using 18-MHz probe in the nasal spine area in a horizontal position. The columellar arteries are found in the paramedian position.

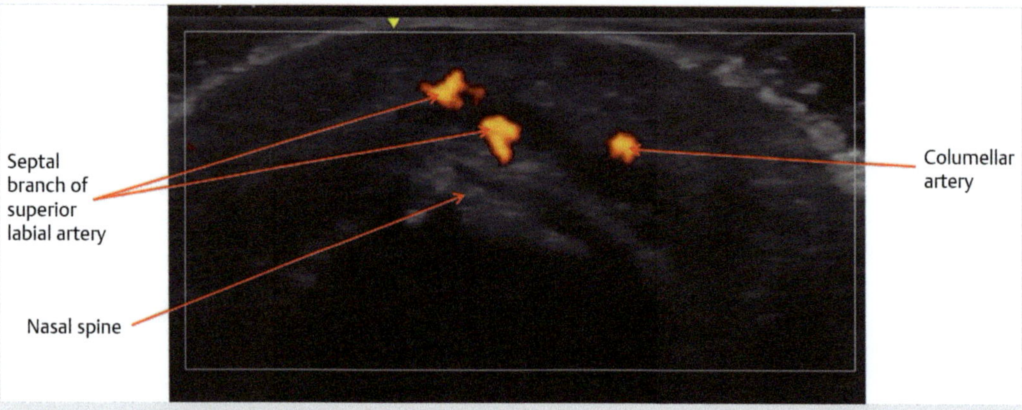

Fig. 3.40 Image obtained using an 18-MHz probe in horizontal orientation underneath nose in nasal spine area. The midline septal branch of the superior labial artery is visualized and this is at risk during injections deep in this area. The columellar artery is paramedian.

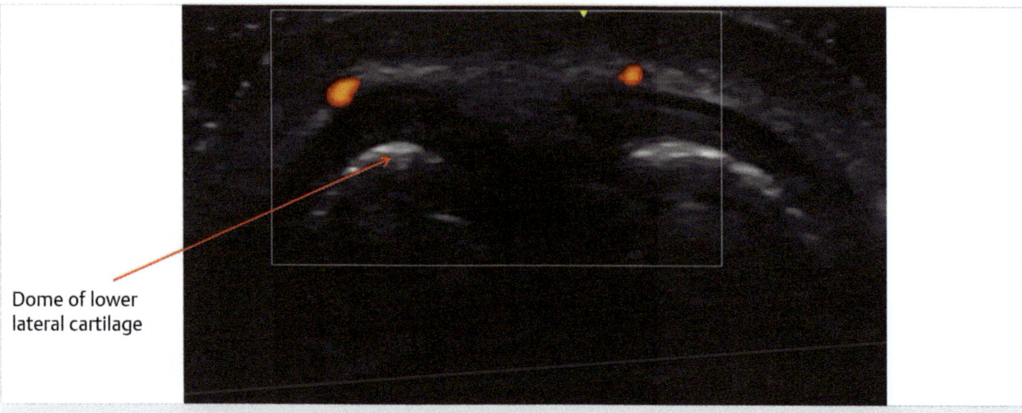

Fig. 3.41 Image obtained with an 18-MHz probe in a horizontal orientation on nasal tip. The arteries probably represent the dorsal nasal arteries but there is an anastomosis of the lateral nasal, dorsal nasal, and columellar arteries in the tip. These arteries are almost uniformly superficial in the tip.

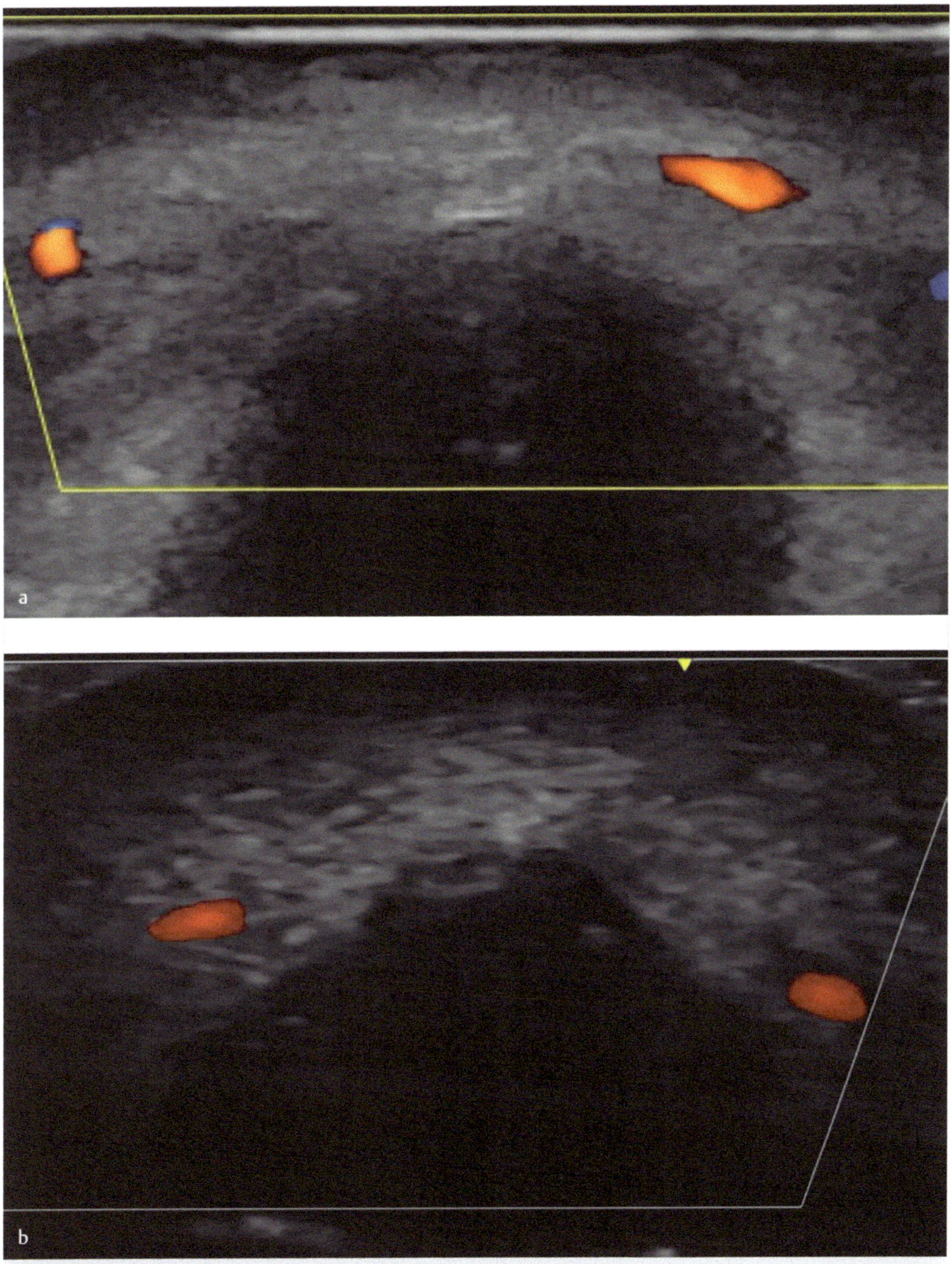

Fig. 3.42 **(a, b)** Upper image obtained using a 20 MHz handheld probe and the lower image with an 18-MHz probe in a horizontal orientation in the mid nasal dorsum. The arteries shown are the dorsal nasal arteries and they are in the usual paramedian position. It is important to visualize the entire dorsum for any midline arteries and their depths.

Suggested Readings

Alfertshofer MG, Frank K, Ehrl D, et al. The layered anatomy of the nose: an ultrasound-based investigation. Aesthet Surg J. 2022; (42)4, Pages 349–357

Beer GM, Manestar M, Mihic-Probst D. The causes of the nasolabial crease: a histomorphological study. Clin Anat. 2013; 26(2): 196–203

Cotofana S, Gotkin RH, Frank K, et al. The functional anatomy of the deep facial fat compartments: a detailed imaging-based investigation. Plast Reconstr Surg. 2019; 143(1):53–63

Cotofana S, Koban KC, Konstantin F, et al. The surface-volume coefficient of the superficial and deep facial fat compartments: a cadaveric three-dimensional volumetric analysis. Plast Reconstr Surg. 2019; 143(6):1605–1613

Desyatnikova S, Barrera P. High-resolution ultrasound for diagnosis and treatment of filler-related septal necrosis. Plastic & Reconstructive Surgery-Global Open. 2024; 12(2): e5630

Gelezhe P, Gombolevskiy V, Morozov S, et al. Three-dimensional description of the angular artery in the nasolabial fold. Aesthet Surg J. 2021; 41(6):697–704

Gierloff M, Stöhring C, Buder T, Gassling V, Açil Y, Wiltfang J. Aging changes of the midfacial fat compartments: a computed tomographic study. Plast Reconstr Surg. 2012; 129(1):263–273

Gierloff M, Stöhring C, Buder T, Wiltfang J. The subcutaneous fat compartments in relation to aesthetically important facial folds and rhytides. J Plast Reconstr Aesthet Surg. 2012; 65 (10):1292–1297

Gombolevskiy V, Gelezhe P, Morozov S, Melnikov DV, et al. The Course of the Angular Artery in the Midface: Implications for Surgical and Minimally Invasive Procedures, Aesthet Surg J. 2021; 41(7):805–813

Karlin J, Vranis N, Dayan E, et al. Post-Hyaluronic Acid Recurrent Eyelid Edema: Pathophysiologic Mechanisms and a Proposed Treatment Protocol, Aesthet Surg J. Open Forum. 2023; (5):ojad102

Lamb J, Surek C. Facial Volumization: An Anatomic Approach. 1st ed. New York, NY: Thieme Medical Publishers; 2017

Lambros V. Facial aging: a 54-year, three-dimensional population study. Plast Reconstr Surg. 2020; 145(4):921–928

Lee W, Kim JS, Moon HJ, Yang EJ. A safe Doppler ultrasound-guided method for nasolabial fold correction with hyaluronic acid filler. Aesthet Surg J. 2021; 41(6):NP486–NP492

Mehta U, Fridirici Z. Advanced techniques in nonsurgical rhinoplasty. Facial Plast Surg Clin North Am. 2019; 27(3):355–365

Mowlds DS, Lambros V. Cheek volumization and the nasolabial fold. Plast Reconstr Surg. 2018; 141(5):1124–1129

Nanayakkara D, Peiris R, Mannapperuma N, Vadysinghe A. Morphometric Analysis of the Infraorbital Foramen: The Clinical Relevance. Anat Res Int. 2016:7917343

Schenck TL, Koban KC, Schlattau A, et al. The functional anatomy of the superficial fat compartments of the face: a detailed imaging study. Plast Reconstr Surg. 2018; 141(6):1351–1359

Siwetz M, Turnowsky N, Hammer N, Pretterklieber M, Wree A, Antipova V. A rare case of facial artery branching—a review of the literature and a case report with clinical implications. Medicina (Kaunas). 2021; 57(11):1172

Surek C. "Facial Anatomy for Filler Injection: The Superficial Musculoaponeurotic System (SMAS) Is Not Just for Facelifting" Clinics in Plastic Surgery. Editors Zins, Charafeddine. Philadelphia, PA. Elsevier

Surek CC, Beut J, Stephens R, Jelks G, Lamb J. Pertinent anatomy and analysis for midface volumizing procedures. Plast Reconstr Surg. 2015; 135(5):818e–829e

Surek C, Beut J, Stephens R, Lamb J, Jelks G. Volumizing viaducts of the midface: defining the Beut techniques. Aesthet Surg J. 2015; 35(2):121–134

Surek CK, Vargo J, Lamb J. Deep pyriform space: anatomical clarifications and clinical implications. Plast Reconstr Surg. 2016; 138 (1):59–64

Tansatit T, Jitaree B, Uruwan S, Rungsawang C. Lower Nose arterial plexus and implications for safe filler injections. Plast Reconstr Surg. 2022 Nov 1;150(5):987e-992e

Wan D, Amirlak B, Giessler P, et al. The differing adipocyte morphologies of deep versus superficial midfacial fat compartments: a cadaveric study. Plast Reconstr Surg. 2014; 133(5): 615e–622e

Walker L, Cetto R. Facial Ageing and Injection Anatomy. 1st ed. UK Book Publishing; 2021

Wong CH, Hsieh MKH, Mendelson B. The tear trough ligament: anatomical basis for the tear trough deformity. Plast Reconstr Surg. 2012; 129(6):1392–1402

Yang HM, Lee JG, Hu KS, et al. New anatomical insights on the course and branching patterns of the facial artery: clinical implications of injectable treatments to the nasolabial fold and nasojugal groove. Plast Reconstr Surg. 2014; 133(5):1077–1082

Chapter 4

Layered Anatomy of the Lower Face

4

4 Layered Anatomy of the Lower Face

Abstract
The lower face contains the deep lateral and deep medial chin fat compartment, the platysma mandibular ligament (PML) and mandibular osseocutaneous retaining ligament (MOCL), and the upper and lower lip anatomical components. This chapter will describe the three-dimensional layering of the lower face, outlining possible targets for injection procedures as well as the vascular anatomy of this region relevant to the clinical injector. Anatomical descriptions are then complemented by detailed ultrasound visuals and technique pearls when imaging the lower face anatomy

Keywords: Platysma muscle, depressor anguli oris muscle, deep lateral chin fat compartment, deep medial cheek fat compartment, platysma mandibular ligament, mandibular osseocutaneous ligament, mentalis muscle, labiomandibular ligament

4.1 Upper and Lower Lip

The cutaneous upper lip and dry vermilion are divided by the "white roll" aka cutaneous–vermilion junction. The white roll is formed by the insertion of the pars marginalis leaflet of the orbicularis oris muscle. Embryologically, the upper lip is formed by two lateral and one central tubercle. The lower lip does not contain a central tubercle but is formed by the fusion to two lateral tubercles at the midline. Recent research has demonstrated compartmentalization of the lip.

The facial artery arises from the neck through the antegonial notch anterior to the masseter muscle. The first branch of the facial artery above the mandibular border is the inferior labial artery (ILA). The ILA demonstrates variation in its patterns and can travel as high as the lower lip vermilion or as low as the mental crease. The ILA often travels at a depth within or just deep to lower lip and chin musculature.

The facial artery continues superiorly and commonly travels approximately 1.5 cm lateral to the oral commissure. The superior labial artery (SLA) is the next branch of the facial artery and initially will travel superior to the white roll and then cross underneath the white roll at depth of approximately 3 cm toward the central tubercle of the upper lip. The SLA terminates as the philtral branch, eventually coursing superiorly to the columella of the nose. The most common depth location of the labial vessels is deep to the orbicularis muscle; however, variation exists where the artery can travel intramuscular or superficial to the muscle (▸ Fig. 4.1, ▸ Fig. 4.2, ▸ Fig. 4.3, ▸ Fig. 4.4).

4.2 Anterior Jawline (Chin, Pre-Jowl, Marionette)

The deep (sub-superficial musculoaponeurotic system [sub-SMAS]) layer in the pre-jowl sulcus contains the deep lateral chin fat compartment. This fat pad is bounded superiorly by the mandibular osseocutaneous ligament (MOCL) and inferiorly by the platysma mandibular ligament (PML). The depressor anguli oris (DAO) is superficial to the deep lateral chin fat compartment (▸ Fig. 4.5, ▸ Fig. 4.6).

The labiomandibular transition is a collection of septations that travel from the DAO to the skin forming the topographic landmark titled the marionette crease. This marks a transition of jowl fat compartment and perioral superficial fat. An analogous structure to the marionette crease is the nasolabial fold. In other words, one could consider the labiomandibular transition and marionette crease as the "nasolabial fold" of the lower lip and pre-jowl region.

Descent of the superficial fat compartments and deflation of the deep fat compartments combined with increased soft tissue laxity over time lead to a deepening of the marionette crease with age. This also creates a "dynamic" muscular strain on the oral commissure and perioral structures that can be visible in multiple phases of perioral animation including smiling and pursing. The deep lateral chin fat compartment is a suitable target for the correction of pre-jowl hollowing. Subcision or discontinuous release of the labiomandibular adhesion can also help soften a harsh or deep marionette shadow, decrease tension on down-turned oral commissures, and create a tissue opening to place filler product between the DAO and skin for volumization. The authors suggest that if using a hyaluronic acid filler in this place to select a rheology that will complement the dynamic movement in the region (▸ Fig. 4.7, ▸ Fig. 4.8, ▸ Fig. 4.9, ▸ Fig. 4.10).

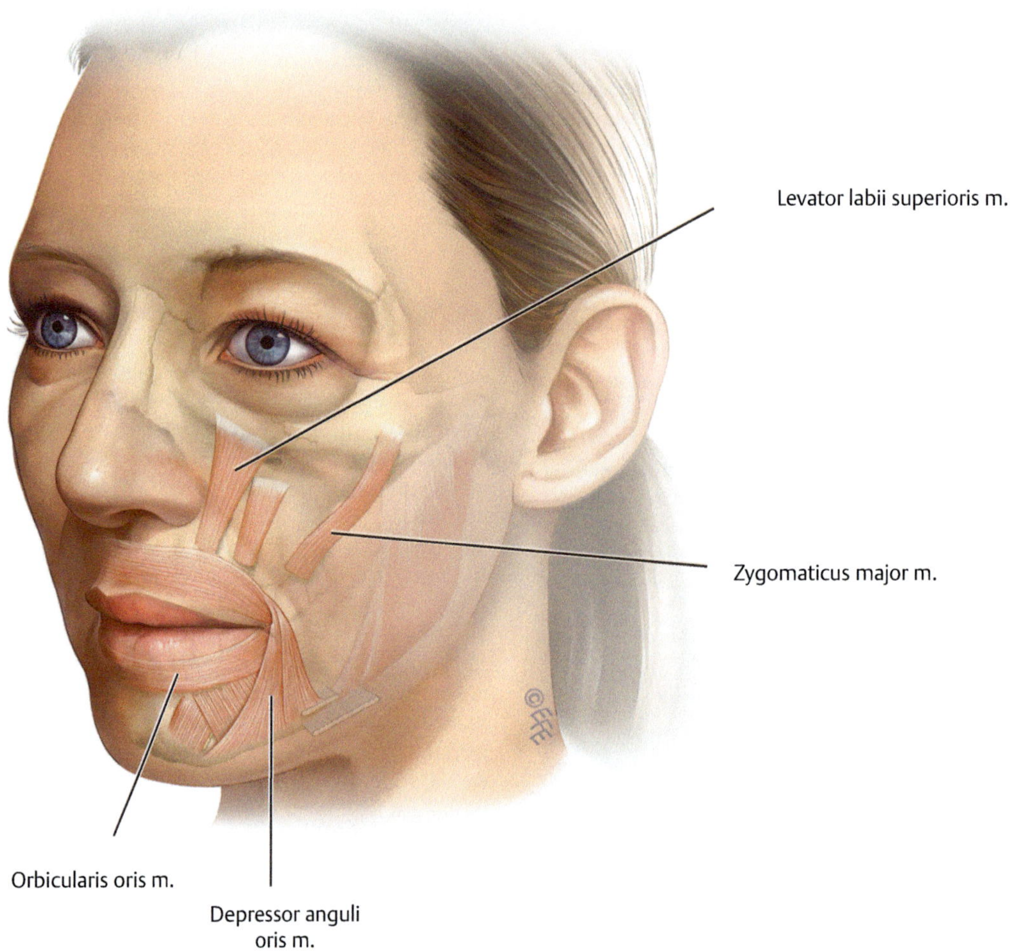

Fig. 4.1 Anatomic illustration of the architecture of the superficial musculoaponeurotic system (SMAS) and muscles of facial expression. © Dr. Levent Efe, CMI.

Key Point

The deep lateral chin fat compartment is a good target for volumization of the pre-jowl sulcus in patients with pre-jowl hollowing. Superficial subcision of the labiomandibular adhesion can soften the marionette crease, decrease dynamic strain in the lower lip perioral subunit, and create a tissue space for deposition of appropriate filler products.

The deep (sub-SMAS) layer in the chin contains the deep medial chin fat compartment which undergoes deflation with age similar to the other deep fat compartments in the face. An important vascular structure in this layer of the chin is the submental artery. The submental artery branches off the facial artery inferior to the mandible and then courses over the periosteum of the menton approximately 6 mm from the midline. The ascending mental artery can have deep and superficial branches, which may anastomose with the inferior labial vasculature. Also, the ascending mental and lingual arteries have direct anastomosis with one another; therefore, vascular occlusions or spasms of the ascending mental artery can manifest as clinical sequelae in the ipsilateral tongue.

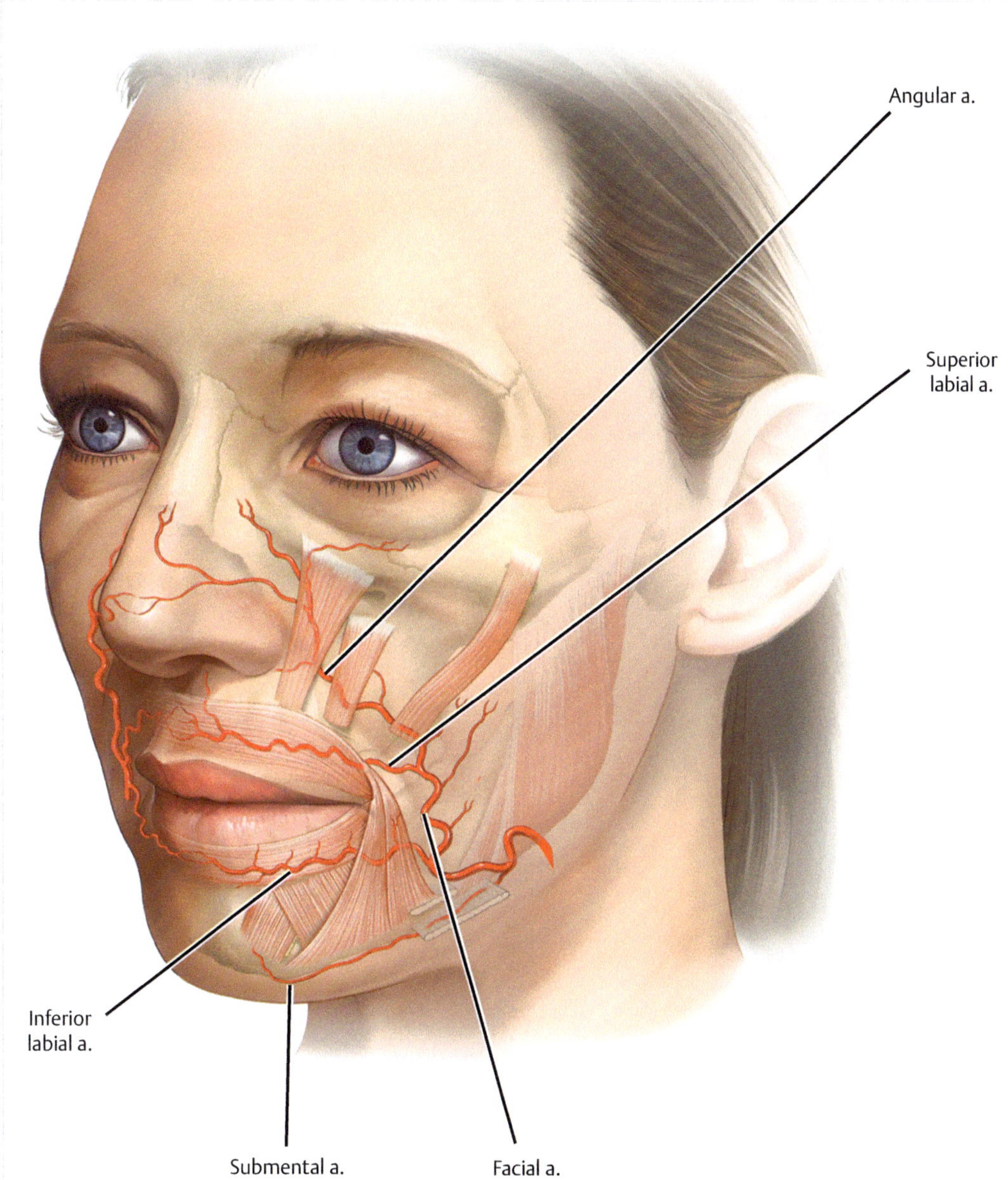

Fig. 4.2 Anatomic illustration of the facial artery and its associated branching patterns. © Dr. Levent Efe, CMI.

The mentalis muscle lies superficial to the deep medial chin fat compartment. Bony resorption and deep fat deflation over time leads to poor support of the fan-shaped mentalis muscle leading to increased muscular strain on the muscle. This is commonly called "mentalis strain" and can manifest as dimpling in the skin overlying the muscle where the fan-shaped fibers of the muscle insert onto the skin. These muscle fibers also contribute to the formation of the labiomental crease (aka mental crease) (▶ Fig. 4.11).

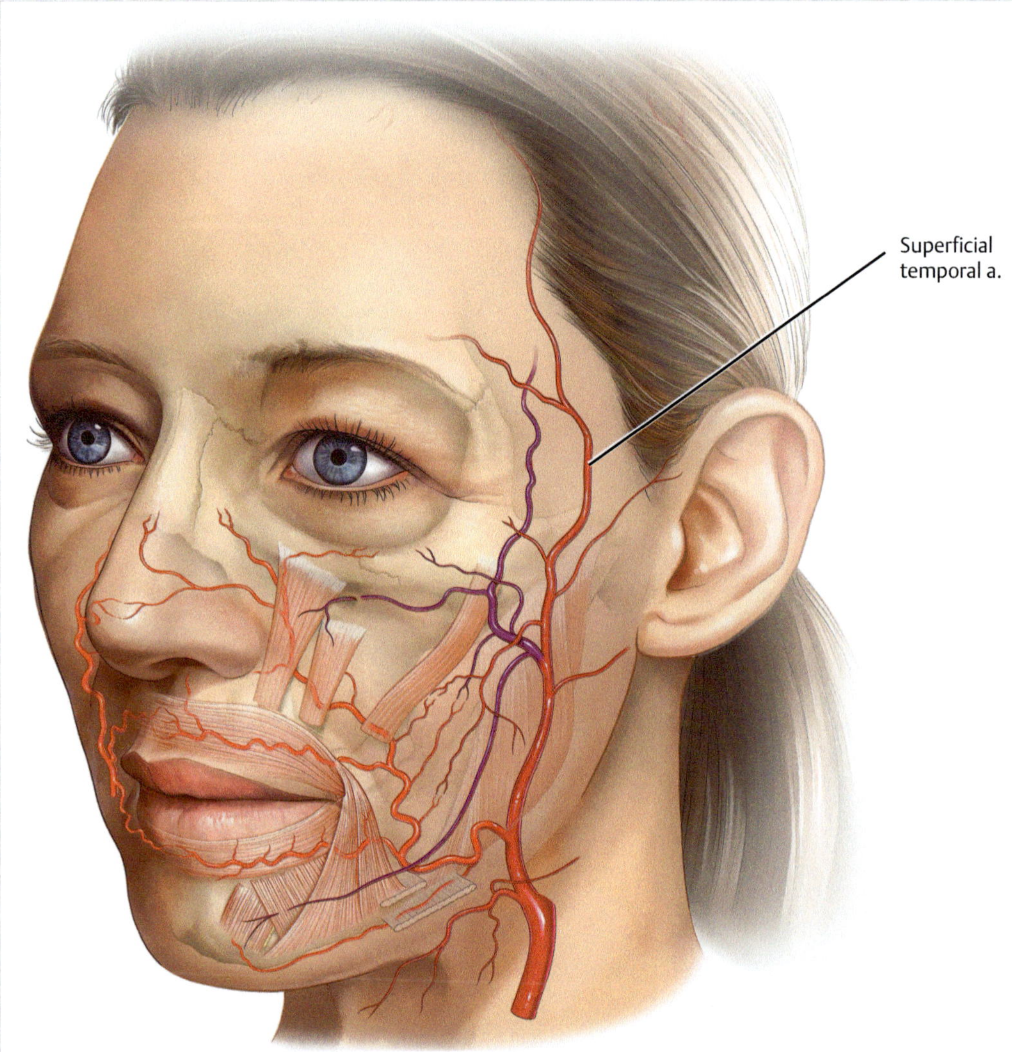

Fig. 4.3 Anatomic illustration of the superficial temporal artery and its associated branching patterns. © Dr. Levent Efe, CMI.

Key Point

"Mentalis strain" can often be caused by lack of deep bony and fat compartment support of the mentalis muscle. When observing mentalis strain clinically, give consideration to restoring deep support of the muscle with targeted volumization into the deep medial chin fat compartment.

4.3 Posterior Jawline

The mandibular ramus and body are the deepest layer in the posterior jawline. The next layer is the masseter muscle, which contains a muscle sling that wraps the lower border of the mandible titled the pterygomasseteric sling. Deep filler injections in this region targeting the periosteum of the mandible often reside in the confines of the masseter muscle and pterygomasseteric sling. Superficial to the masseter muscle lies the parotid gland, which

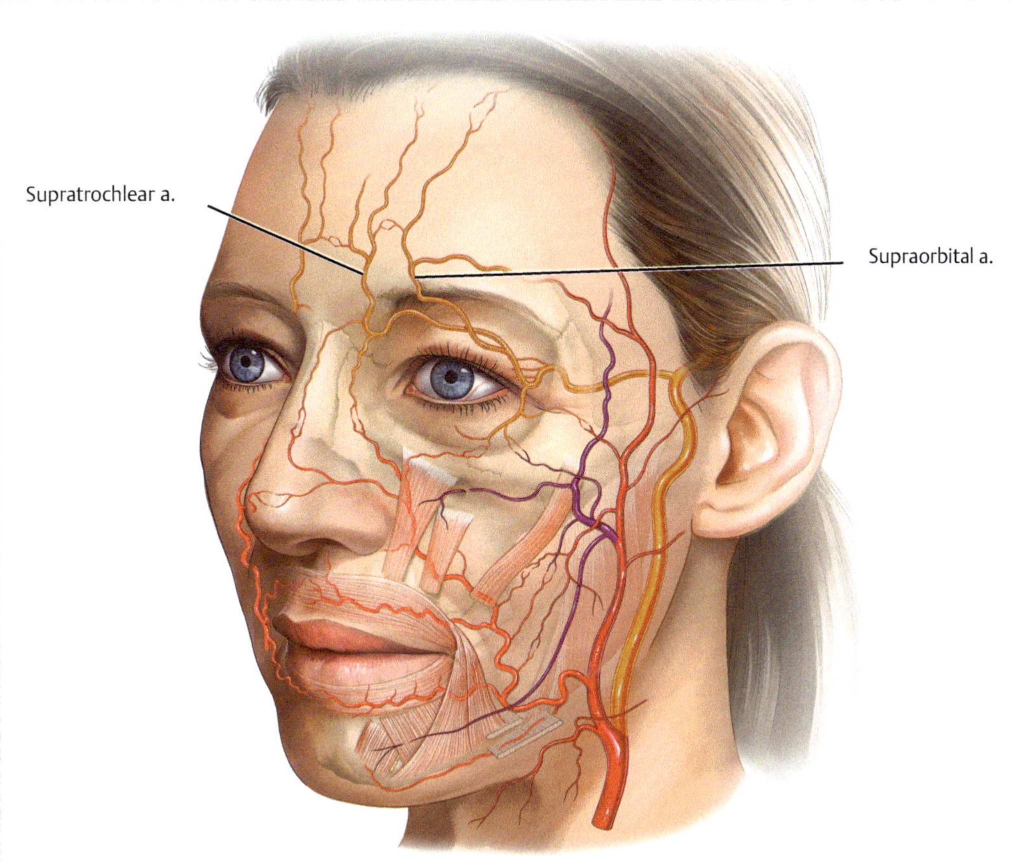

Fig. 4.4 Anatomic illustration of the supratrochlear and supraorbital arteries and their associated branching patterns. © Dr. Levent Efe, CMI.

is covered by the parotid capsule. The platysma muscle courses superficial to the parotid capsule coalescing with the SMAS in the face. Superficial to the platysma and SMAS lies the superficial lateral cheek fat compartment. This fibrofatty compartment can serve as a suitable target for superficial (supra-SMAS) injections for posterior jawline sculpting and contouring (▶ Fig. 4.12).

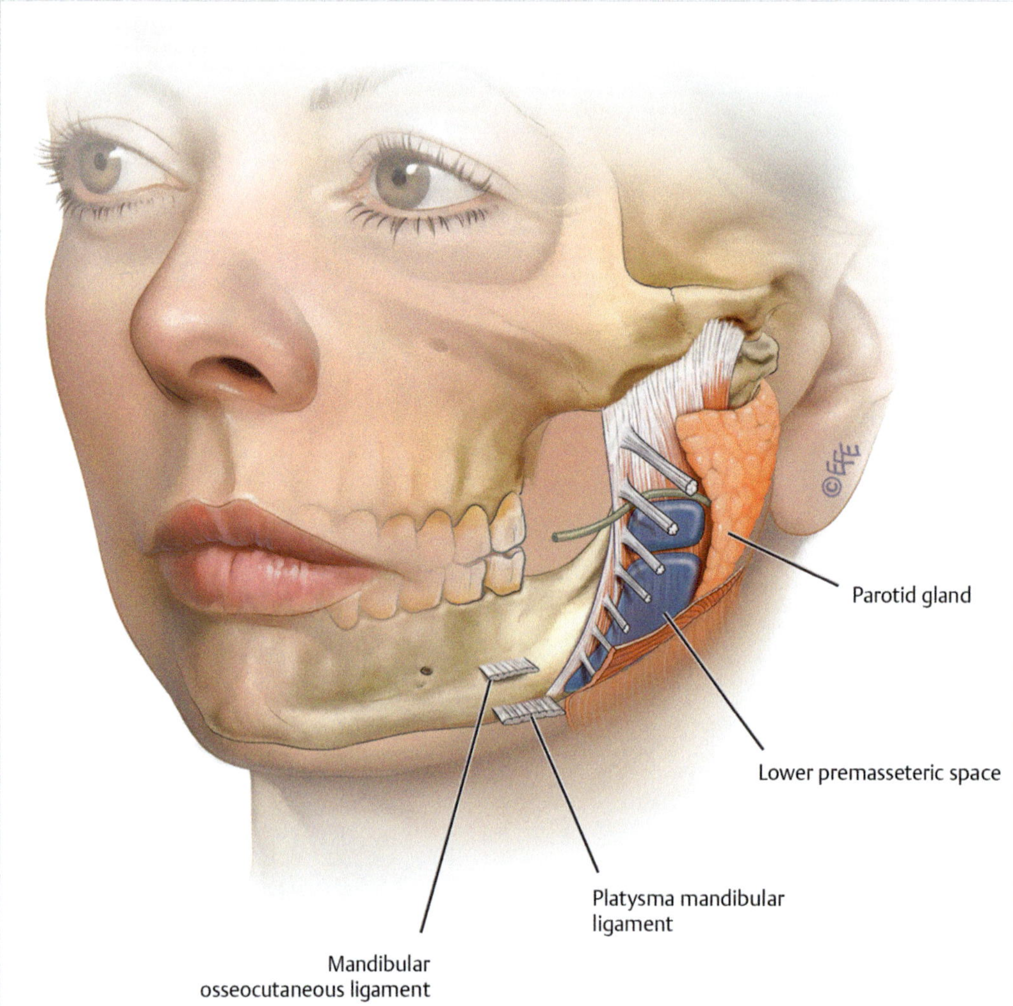

Fig. 4.5 Anatomic illustration of the jawline, pre-jowl sulcus, and marionette, demonstrating the parotid gland, lower premasseteric space, and masseteric retaining ligaments. Note the mandibular osseocutaneous retaining ligament and platysmal mandibular retaining ligament which form the superior and inferior boundary of the pre-jowl sulcus (aka deep lateral chin fat compartment). © Dr. Levent Efe, CMI.

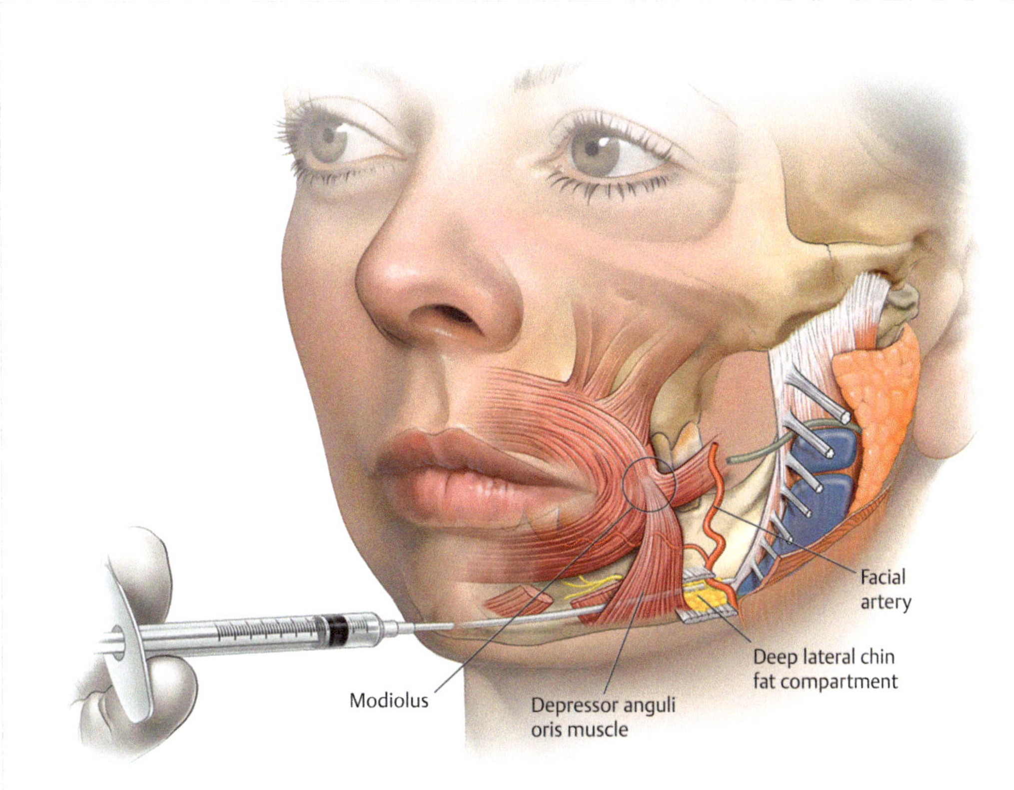

Fig. 4.6 Anatomic illustration of the pre-jowl sulcus and marionette, demonstrating the facial artery descending through the antegonial notch and running within the depressor anguli oris (DAO) which is synonymous with the superficial musculoaponeurotic system (SMAS). The deep lateral chin fat compartment resides between the platysmal mandibular ligament (PML) and mandibular osseocutaneous ligament (MOCL). © Dr. Levent Efe, CMI.

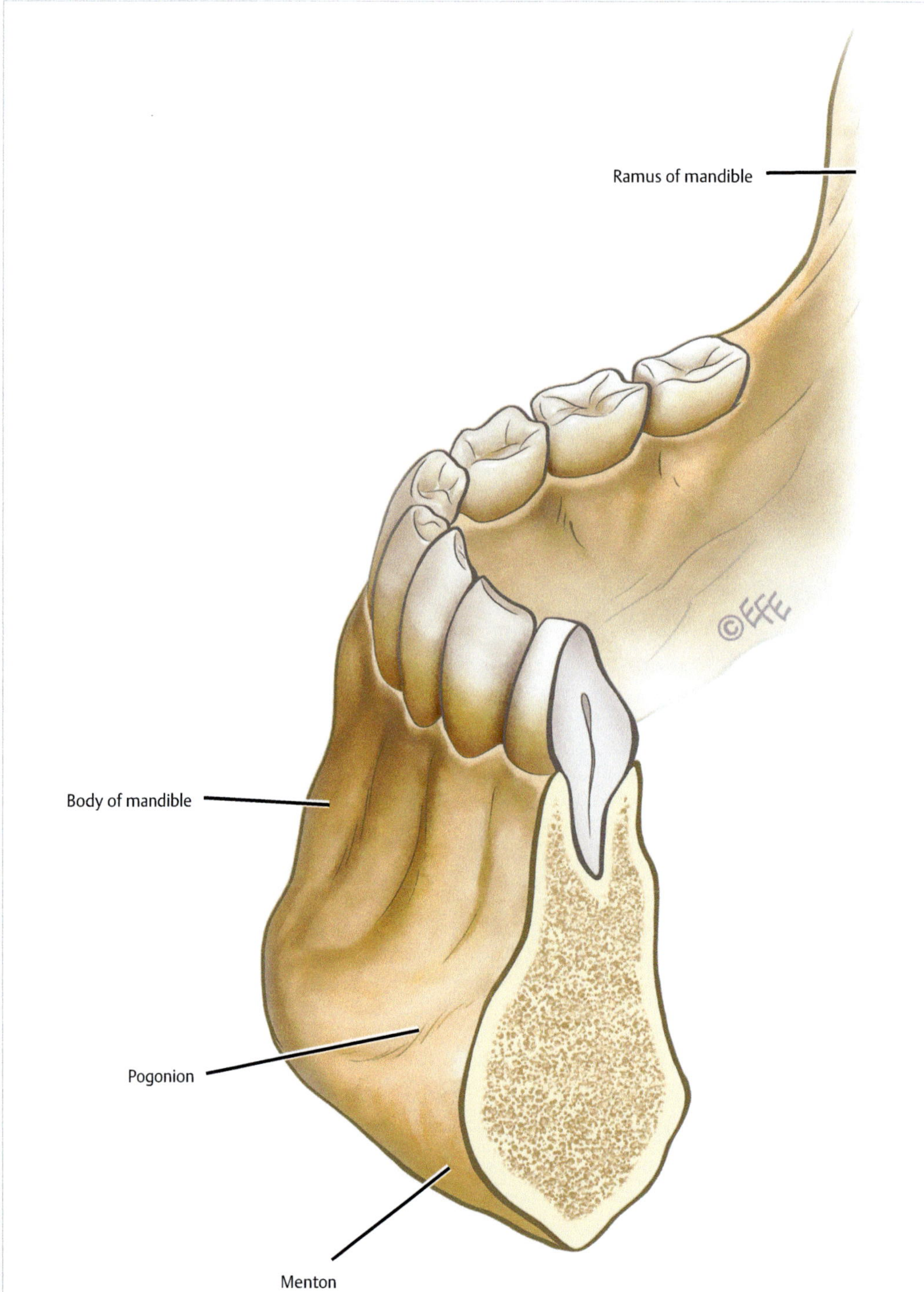

Fig. 4.7 Anatomic illustration of the anterior jawline and chin demonstrating the mandibular body, mentum, and dentition. © Dr. Levent Efe, CMI.

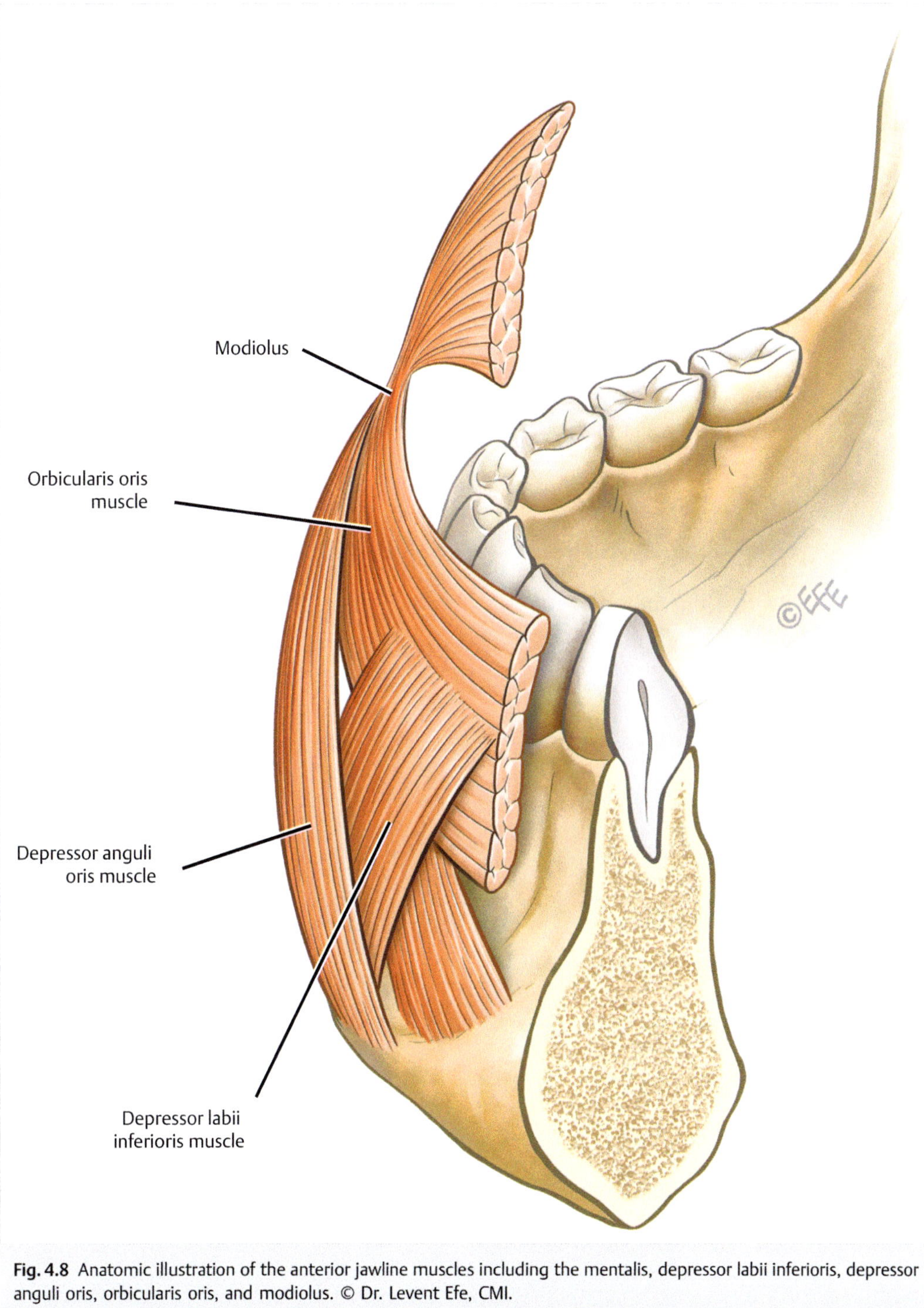

Fig. 4.8 Anatomic illustration of the anterior jawline muscles including the mentalis, depressor labii inferioris, depressor anguli oris, orbicularis oris, and modiolus. © Dr. Levent Efe, CMI.

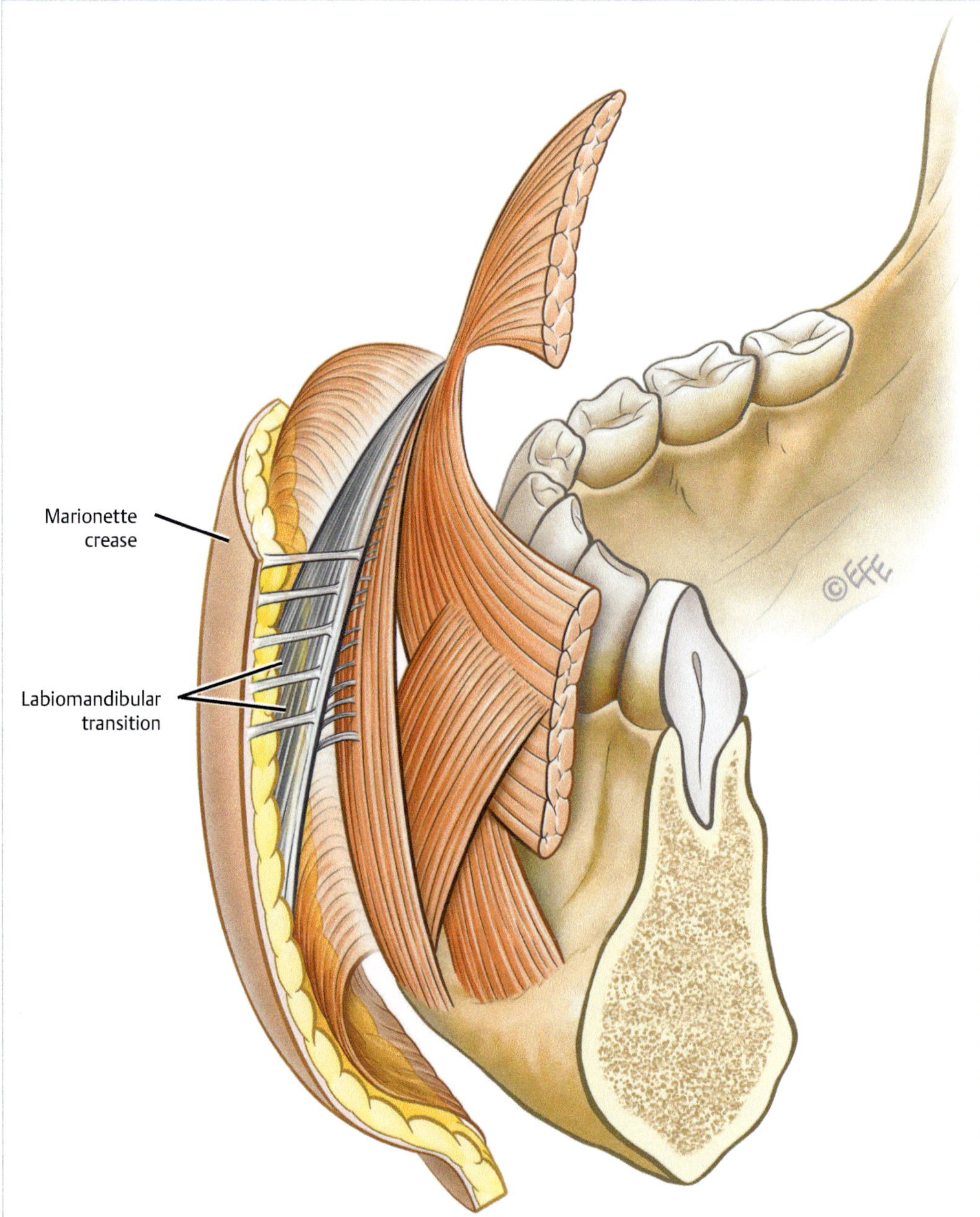

Fig. 4.9 Anatomic illustration of the septations between the lip depressors and the skin forming the topographic landmark of the marionette crease. © Dr. Levent Efe, CMI.

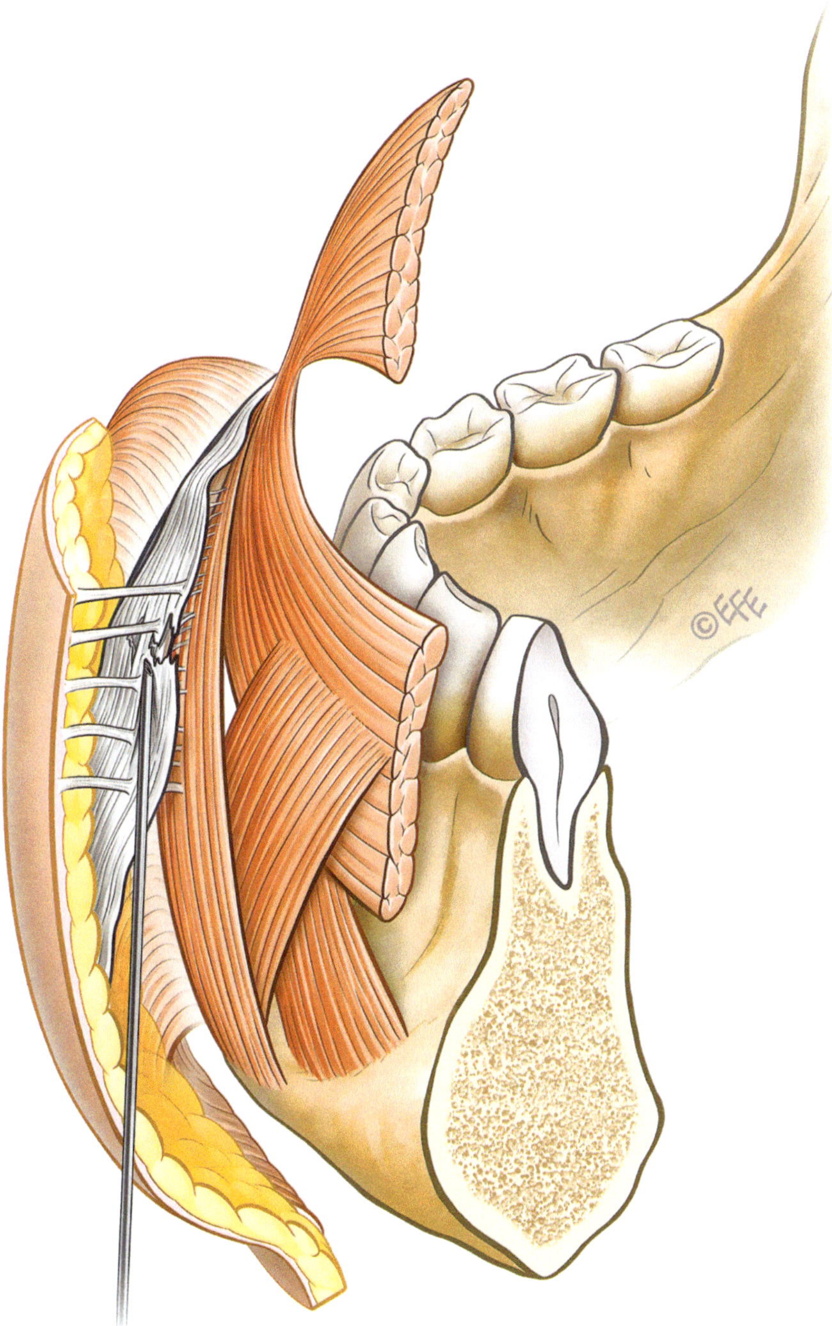

Fig. 4.10 Anatomic illustration of the anatomic disruption of the marionette crease utilizing subcision technique. © Dr. Levent Efe, CMI.

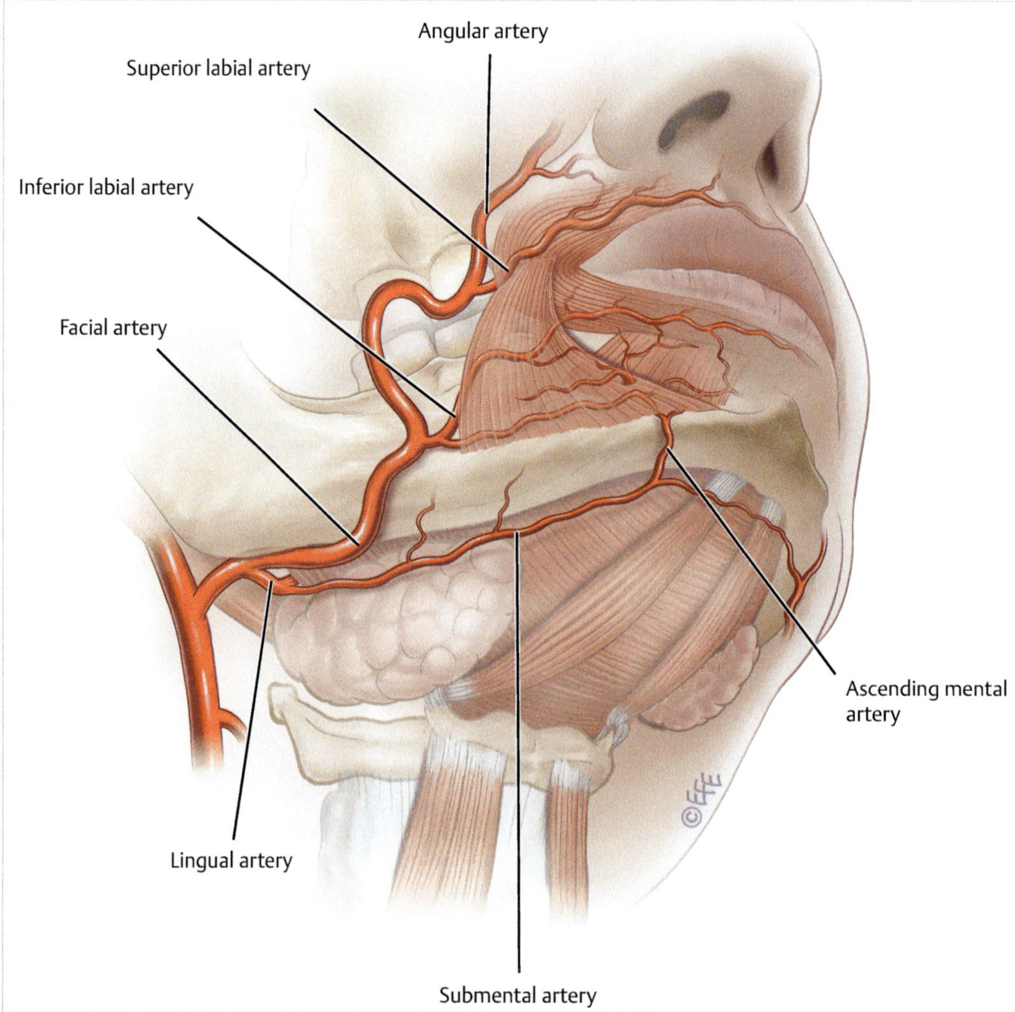

Fig. 4.11 Anatomic illustration of the vasculature of the anterior jawline, marionette, and chin. The ascending mental artery shares a common arterial trunk with the lingual artery. There can be vascular anastomotic connection between the inferior labial artery and ascending mental arteries. The ascending mental artery commonly travels over the mentum paramidline. © Dr. Levent Efe, CMI.

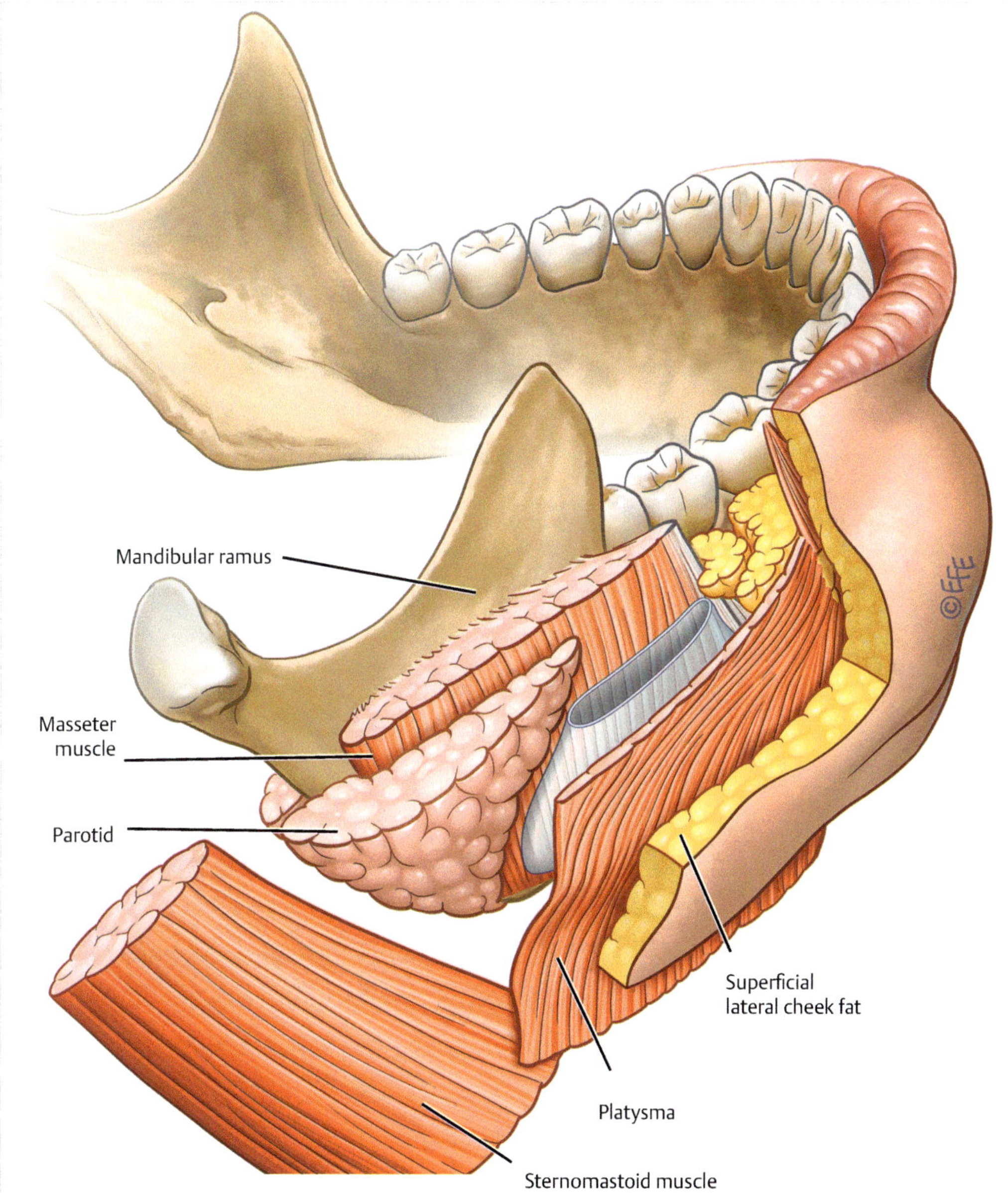

Fig. 4.12 Anatomic illustration of the posterior jawline demonstrating the mandibular ramus, masseter muscle, parotid gland and capsule, platysma muscle, and superficial lateral cheek fat. © Dr. Levent Efe, CMI.

4.4 Ultrasound Anatomy and Technique for the Lower Face

Within the lower face, ultrasound imaging demonstrates the highly variable vascular anatomy of the superior and inferior labial, and the angular arteries. There are several patterns repeated such as the relationship of the facial artery being lateral to the DAO muscle and the mental foramen lying deep to the DAO. The labial arteries are highly variable, lying deep, within, or superficial to the orbicularis oris muscle, with the inferior labial being more tortuous and less predictable. The ascending branches of the submental artery can be low flow and < 1 mm in diameter so gain must be turned up and velocity scale turned down for best visualization. Often power Doppler is a better mode to use for these vessels (▶ Fig. 4.13, ▶ Fig. 4.14, ▶ Fig. 4.15, ▶ Fig. 4.16, ▶ Fig. 4.17, ▶ Fig. 4.18, ▶ Fig. 4.19, ▶ Fig. 4.20, ▶ Fig. 4.21, ▶ Fig. 4.22, ▶ Fig. 4.23, ▶ Fig. 4.24, ▶ Fig. 4.25, ▶ Fig. 4.26, ▶ Fig. 4.27, ▶ Fig. 4.28, ▶ Fig. 4.29, ▶ Fig. 4.30, ▶ Fig. 4.31, ▶ Fig. 4.32, ▶ Fig. 4.33, ▶ Fig. 4.34, ▶ Fig. 4.35, ▶ Fig. 4.36, ▶ Fig. 4.37, ▶ Fig. 4.38, ▶ Fig. 4.39).

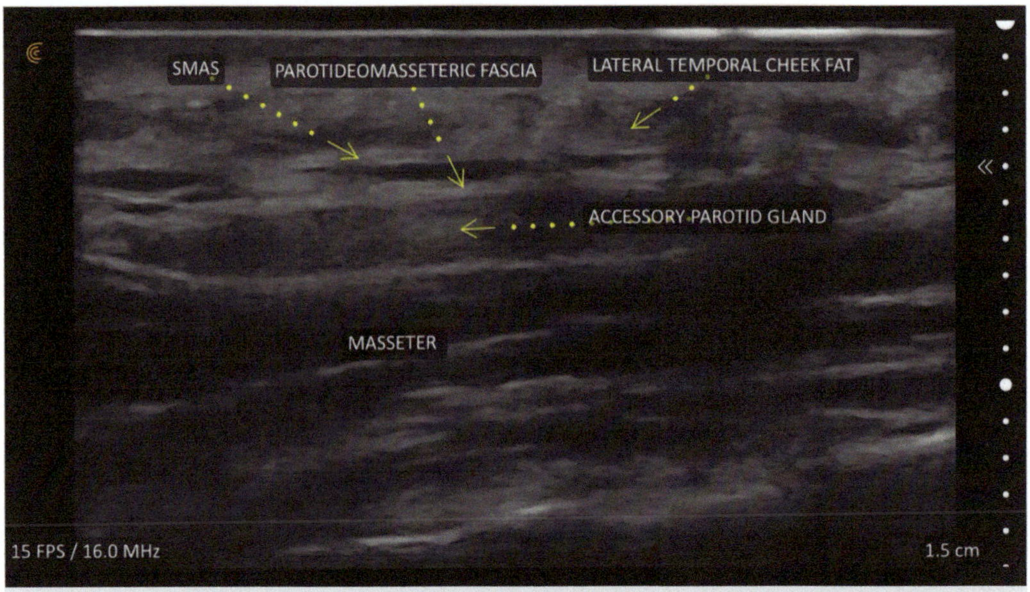

Fig. 4.13 Image obtained using a 20-MHz handheld probe in a horizontal position. An accessory parotid gland lies anterior to the parotid gland near the course of the parotid duct on the lateral aspect of the masseter. The parotideomasseteric fascia overlies the parotid and masseter and is considered "deep fascia" and inserts superior into the lower border of the zygomatic arch. A more superficial fascial layer is the superficial musculoaponeurotic system (SMAS). Superficial to the SMAS is the lateral cheek fat (lateral temporal cheek fat). The incidence of an accessory parotid gland ranges from 7.5 – 56%.

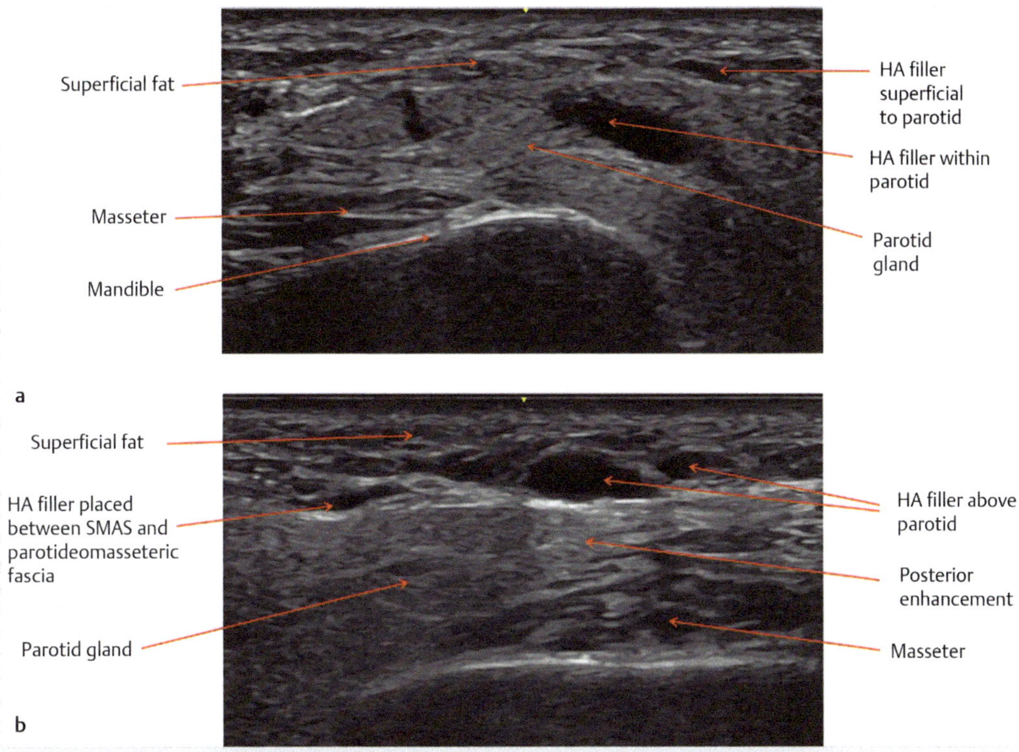

Fig. 4.14 (**a**) Image obtained using an 18-MHz probe in horizontal position in preauricular area. This image shows hyaluronic acid (HA) filler within the parotid gland and HA filler superficial to the gland. Injections into the submalar and preauricular area must be placed in this superficial fat layer to avoid parotid complications. (**b**) Image obtained using 18-MHz probe in horizontal orientation in the preauricular area. There is HA filler in between the two fascial layers on the left side of image. On the right side of the image is HA placed in the subcutaneous fat and the preferred plane by the authors (SW and CS). Posterior enhancement is a commonly seen artifact posterior to a pocket of HA.

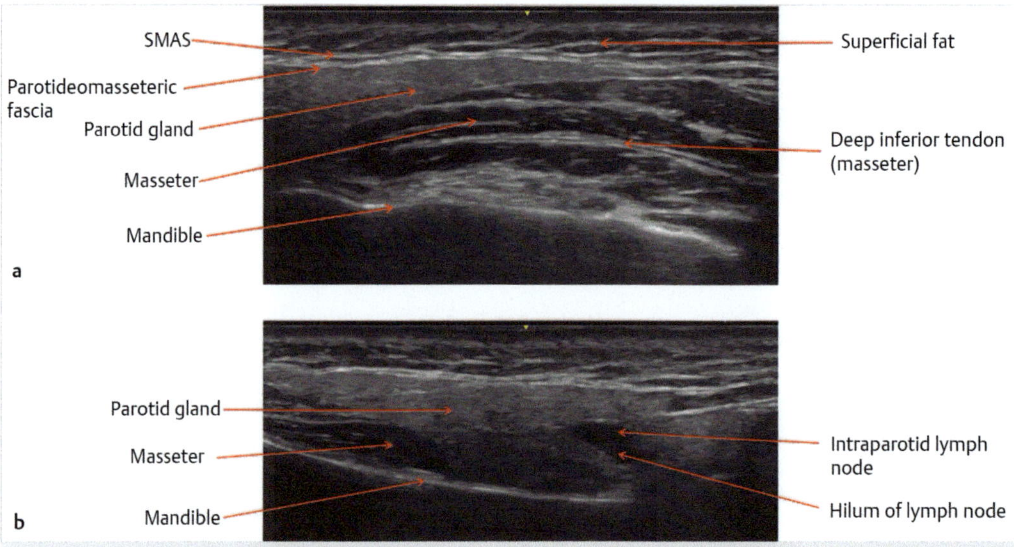

Fig. 4.15 (a) Image obtained with a 20-MHz probe in horizontal position in pre-auricular area. The superficial fat in this area is the preferred target of filler by the authors (SW and CS). It is a small space which can measure 1-3 mm in depth. Injections can inadvertently enter the parotid by piercing the SMAS and parotideomasseteric fascia with little to no discomfort to the patient during the procedure. Complications such as swelling, pain, infection, sialocele can occur as a result. (**b**) Image obtained with a 20-MHz probe in vertical orientation in the right preauricular area. A lymph node is found within the parotid as a hypoechoic structure (HA filler is anechoic). It also has a distinct hilum, an isoechoic structure which is where the vessels, including lymphatic vessels drain from the lymph node medulla. Power doppler can be used to see vascularity of the hilum.

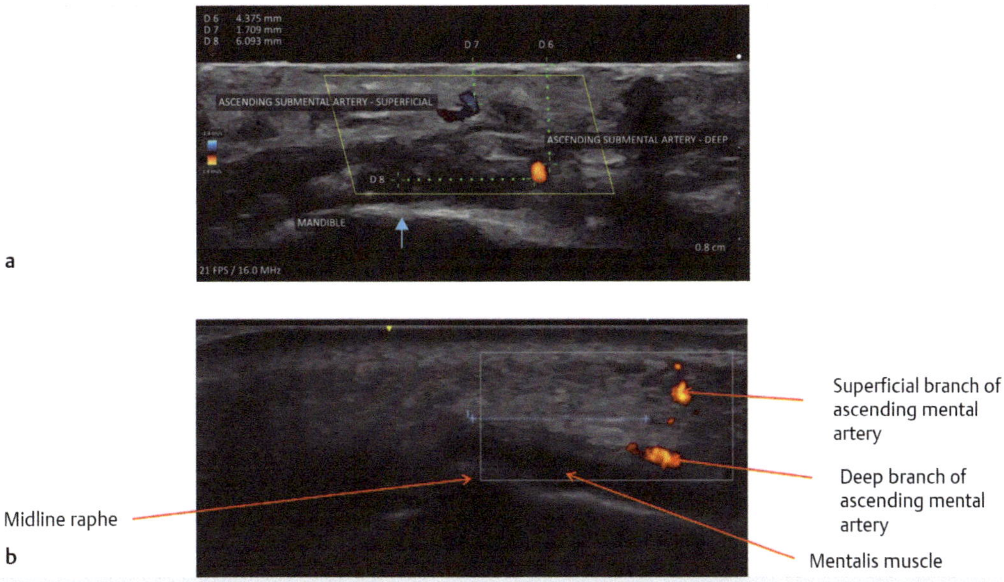

Fig. 4.16 (**a**) Image obtained using a 20-MHz probe in a horizontal position on the left side. The submental artery arises from the facial artery below the mandibular border. It travels medially and crosses over the border paramedially, at an average of 6 mm (D 8) from the midline (blue arrow). There is usually a superficial and a deep ascending submental artery (also named the ascending mental artery). This artery anastomoses with the mental, inferior labial, and with the lingual artery via the sublingual artery. There are cases of hemi-tongue occlusions from filler injections in the chin. (**b**) Image obtained using a 20-MHz probe in horizontal orientation using power doppler mode. In this patient, the deep branch of the ascending mental artery is 9 mm from the midline with the superficial branch slightly more lateral. Power doppler is mode of choice for this low flow artery (SW).

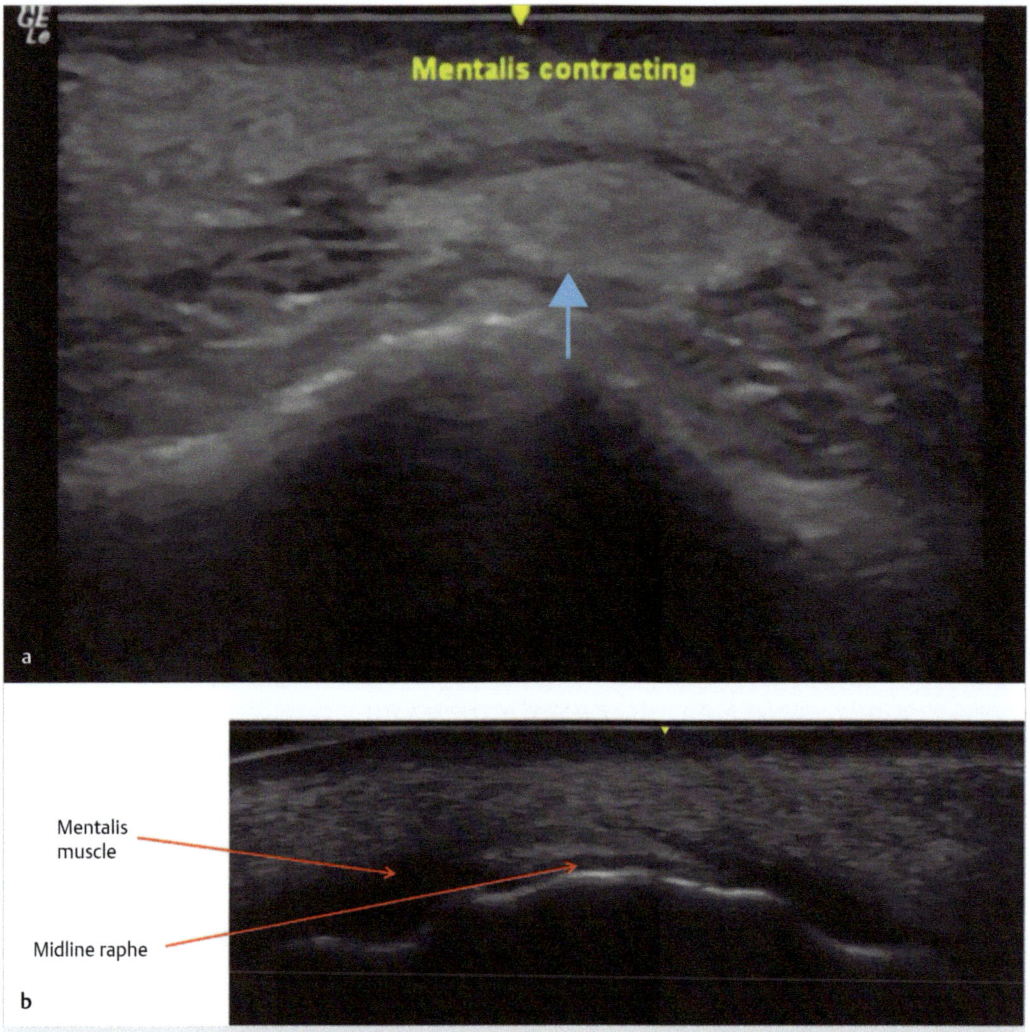

Fig. 4.17 (**a**) Image obtained using an 18-MHz probe in horizontal position. The mentalis is a midline muscle that has a midline tendinous thickening at its origin which can lead to patient discomfort during cannula filler enhancement. The insertion of the mentalis muscle is in the mentolabial sulcus (chin crease). (**b**) Image obtained using a 20-MHz probe in a horizontal orientation over the chin. The midline raphe can be seen with the mentalis muscle on either side of it.

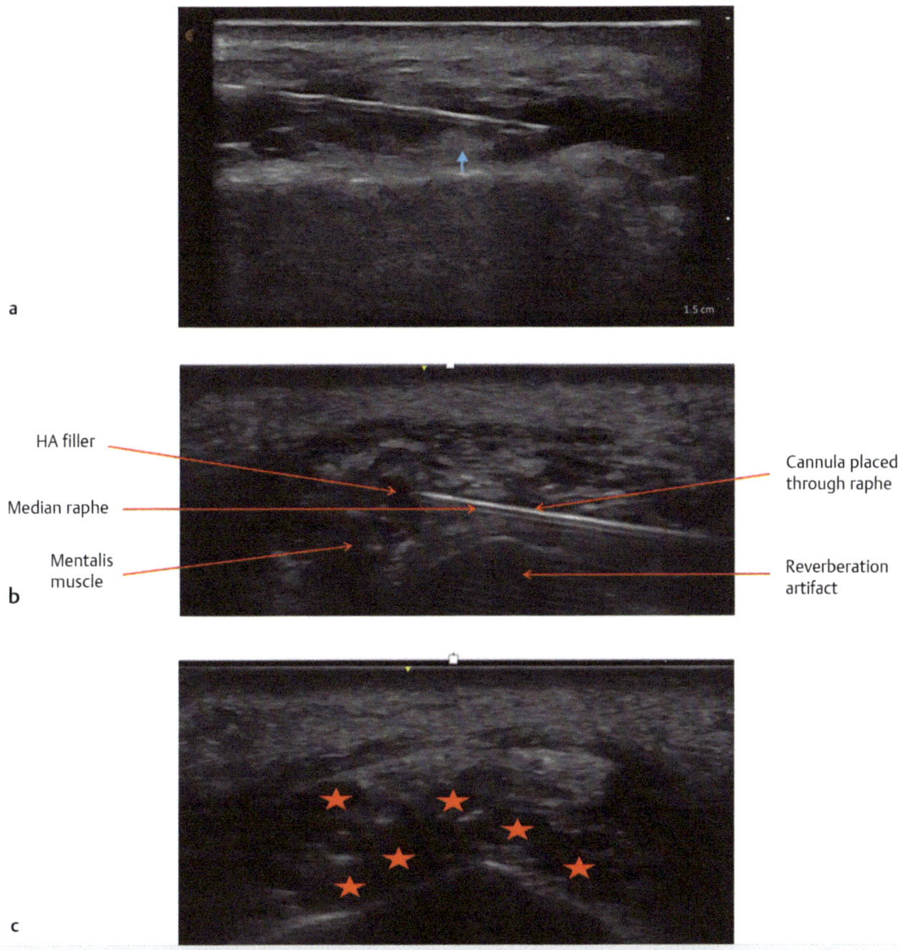

Fig. 4.18 (**a**) Image obtained using a 20-MHz probe in horizontal position. Cannula is seen crossing through the midline tendinous attachment of the mentalis muscle (blue arrow) and injecting hyaluronic acid (HA) filler along the periosteum. (**b**) Image obtained using the 18-MHz probe in horizontal orientation over the chin. The cannula is seen passing through the median raphe of the chin. This technique is the preferred method of the author (SW) for its safety aspects. This technique also limits the backflow of filler along the cannula. (**c**) Image shows the results of the cannula technique with the stars representing HA filler. Reverberation artifact is seen posterior to a cannula or needle and can be used by the injector as a means of "finding" the cannula/needle during guided injections.

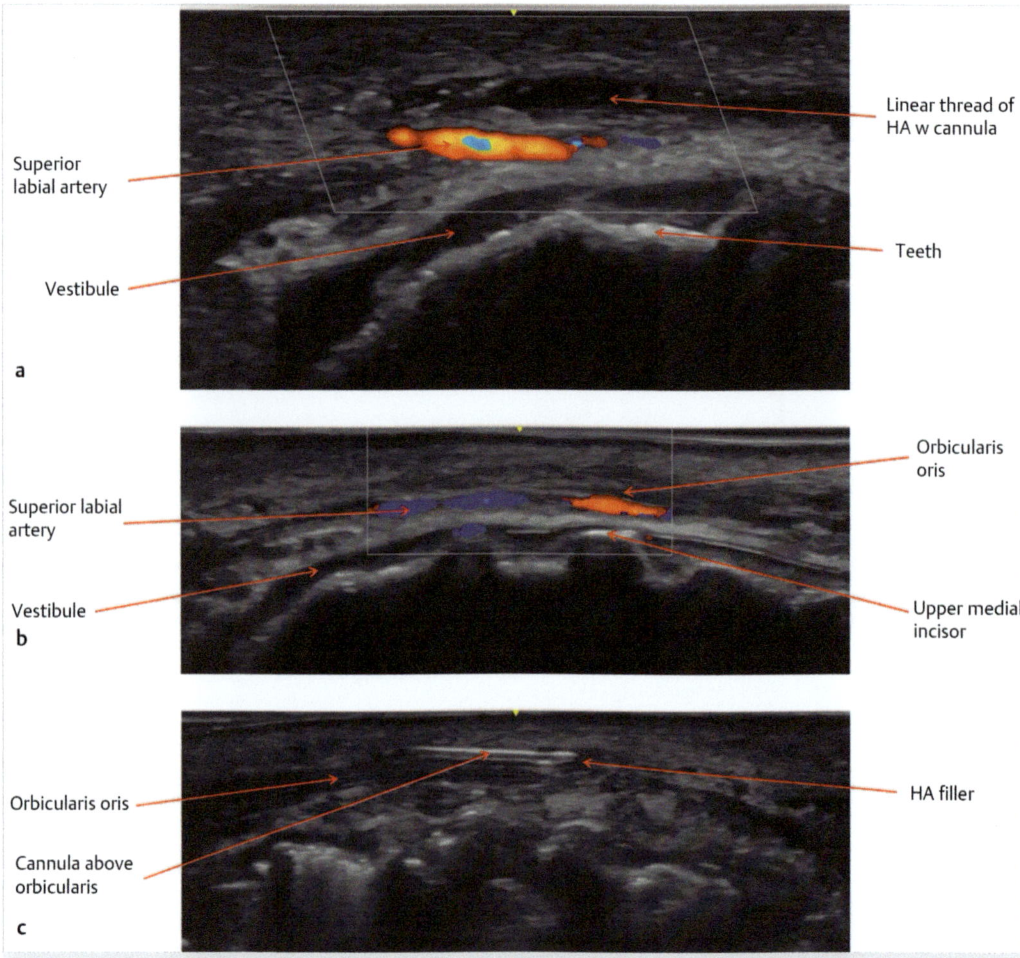

Fig. 4.19 **(a)** Image is obtained using an 18-MHz probe in a horizonal orientation on upper lip. This is immediately after filler placement with cannula in the submucosa, superficial to the superior labial artery. The anechoic vestibule is often confused with the orbicularis oris muscle but can be discerned from that by having the patient place their tongue between their teeth and lip. **(b)** Image obtained using an 18-MHz probe in a horizontal position on the upper lip. The superior labial artery lies in its typical position just deep to the orbicularis oris. The upper and lower lip can be differentiated by the size of the medial incisors with the upper teeth being larger. **(c)** Image obtained using an 18-MHz probe in a horizontal position on the lower lip. The cannula is seen superficial to the orbicularis oris muscle. Note the medial incisors are smaller than the upper medial incisors.

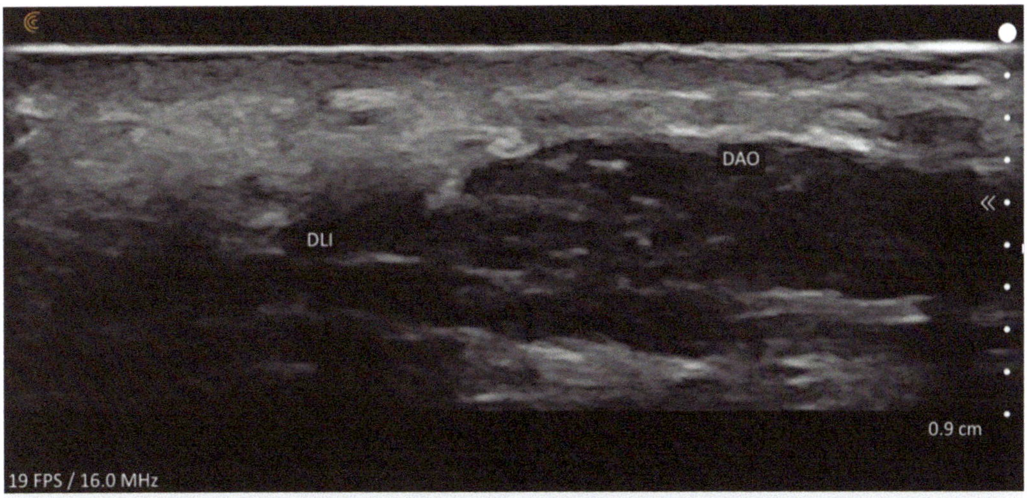

Fig. 4.20 Image obtained using a 20-MHz handheld probe in horizontal position on the left side of face. This image shows the relationship between the depressor anguli oris (DAO) and the depressor labii inferioris (DLI). The DAO is lateral and superficial to the DLI. The DAO is undergoing contraction in this image (frowning). The DAO is a larger muscle than the DLI. Of note, the two muscles overlap and to avoid inadvertent neurotoxin spread to the DLI when injecting DAO muscle, it is recommended to inject the DAO inferiorly, laterally, and superficially. The DAO origin is just anterior to the masseter muscle.

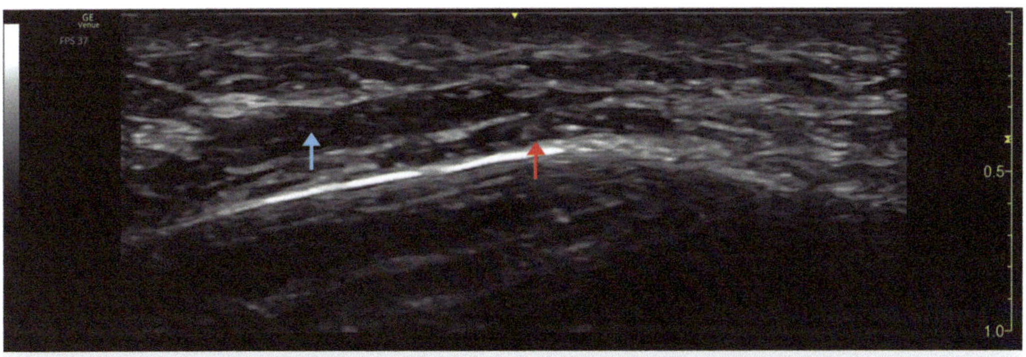

Fig. 4.21 Image obtained using an 18-MHz probe in horizontal plane on left side. The depressor anguli oris (DAO) muscle (blue arrow) is seen as a thicker muscle that lies superficial to the depressor labii inferioris (DLI) muscle. Note the overlap of the two muscles puts the DLI at risk during neurotoxin injections. This overlap is variable and can be nearly half of the DAO. The thickness of the two muscles is variable as well and seems to be less in the younger patients (this patient is 19 years old).

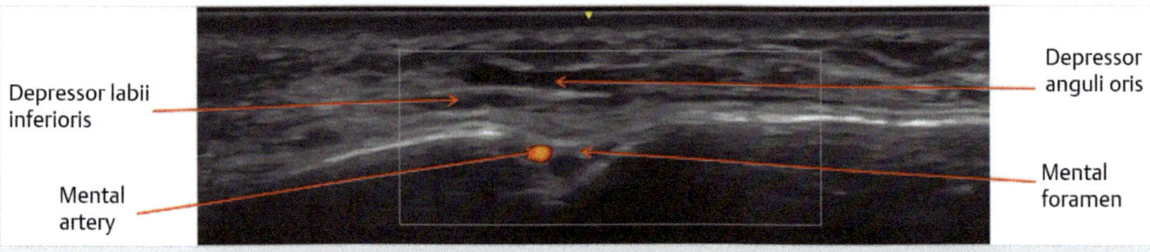

Fig. 4.22 Image obtained using a 20-MHz probe in a horizontal position in left marionette area. Visible in the image is the mental artery within the mental foramen. There is significant overlap of the depressor labii inferioris (DLI) and depressor anguli oris (DAO) muscles in this image. The overlap of these two muscles puts the DLI at risk during injections in the DAO. It is the author's (SW) preferred injection technique to inject the DAO laterally, inferiorly, and superficially to avoid spread to the DLI. Note the DAO is a bigger muscle than the DLI muscle.

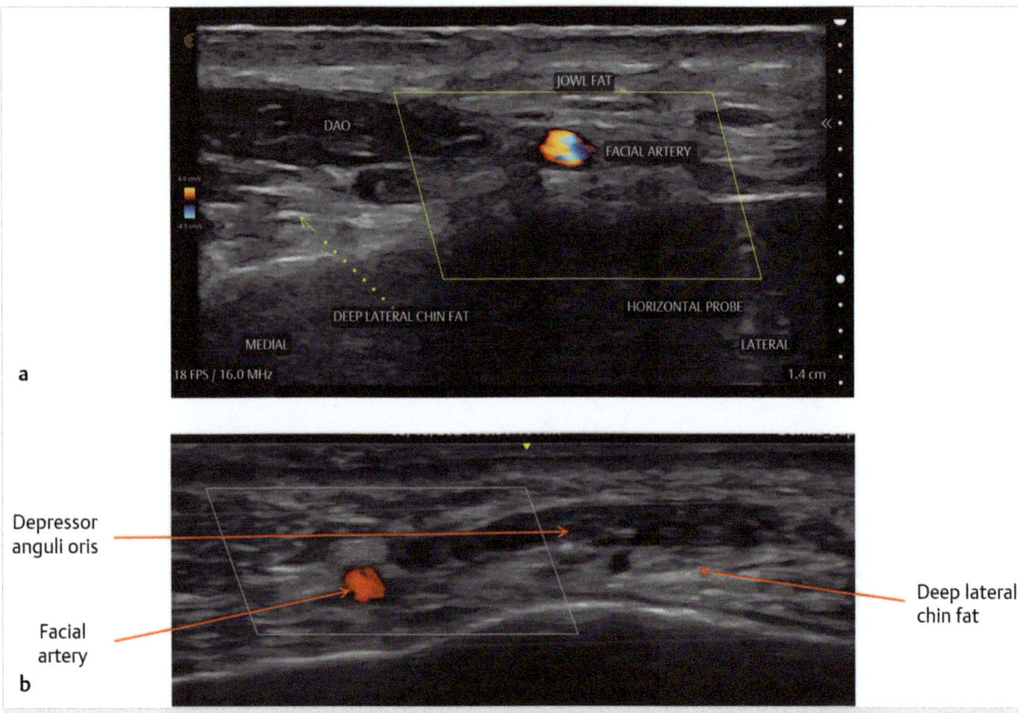

Fig. 4.23 (**a**) Image obtained using a 20-MHz handheld horizontal probe, left side. This image shows the constant relationship of the facial artery lying lateral to the depressor anguli oris (DAO) muscle. Superficial and lateral to DAO is the jowl fat (superficial fat pad). Lying deep to the DAO is the deep lateral chin fat. (**b**) Image obtained using a 20-MHz probe in horizontal orientation in the marionette area on the patient's right. Facial artery seen just posterior to the DAO and the deep lateral chin fat is deep to the DAO.

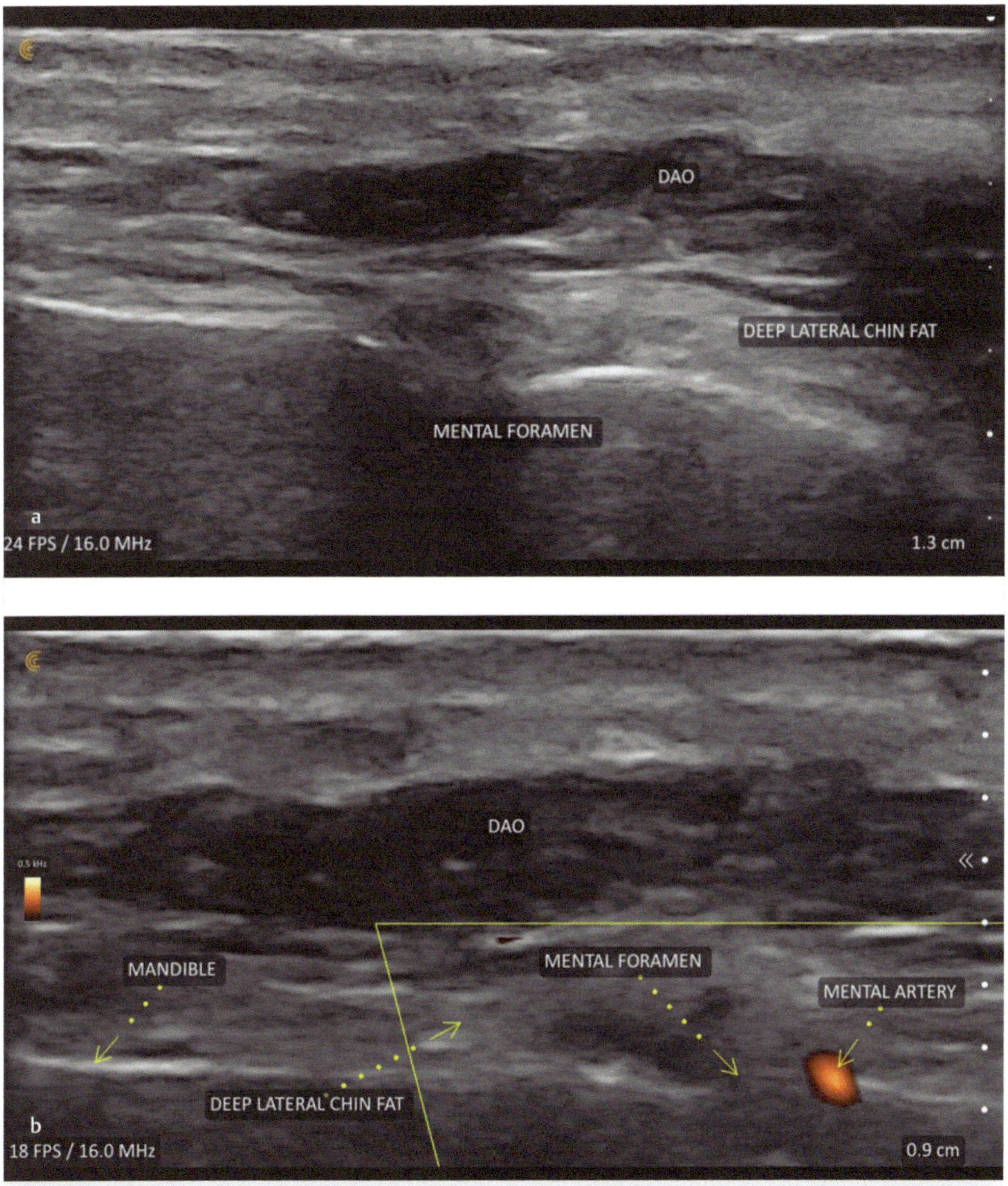

Fig. 4.24 (**a, b**) Image obtained using a 20-MHz probe in horizontal position. The depressor anguli oris (DAO) is a fairly distinct ultrasound landmark. Deep to the DAO is the deep lateral chin fat and the mental foramen. Contained within the mental foramen is the mental artery and nerve. The mental artery is usually difficult to image so power Doppler mode is often required. The mental foramen can be rapidly identified by searching for a discontinuity in the mandible.

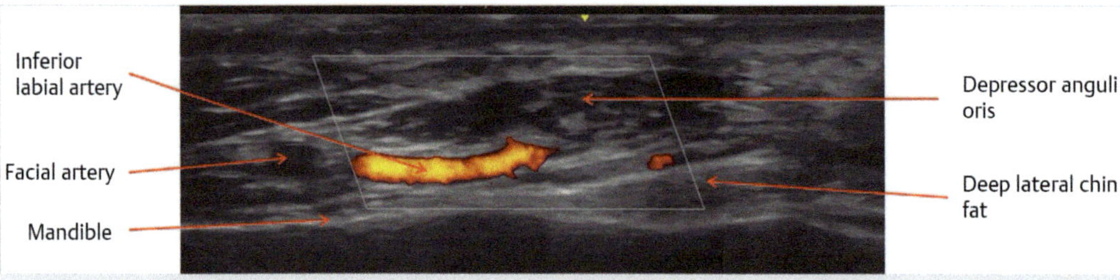

Fig. 4.25 Image obtained using a 20-MHz probe in horizontal position in marionette area. The inferior labial artery is deep (ILA) to the depressor anguli oris (DAO) and can be found as low as the mental crease. Occasionally, there is a variant artery called a labiomental artery, which is a branch of the facial artery that takes off before the ILA. The deep lateral chin fat compartment is always deep to the depressor anguli oris (DAO) and is partially responsible for the volume loss in the marionette crease.

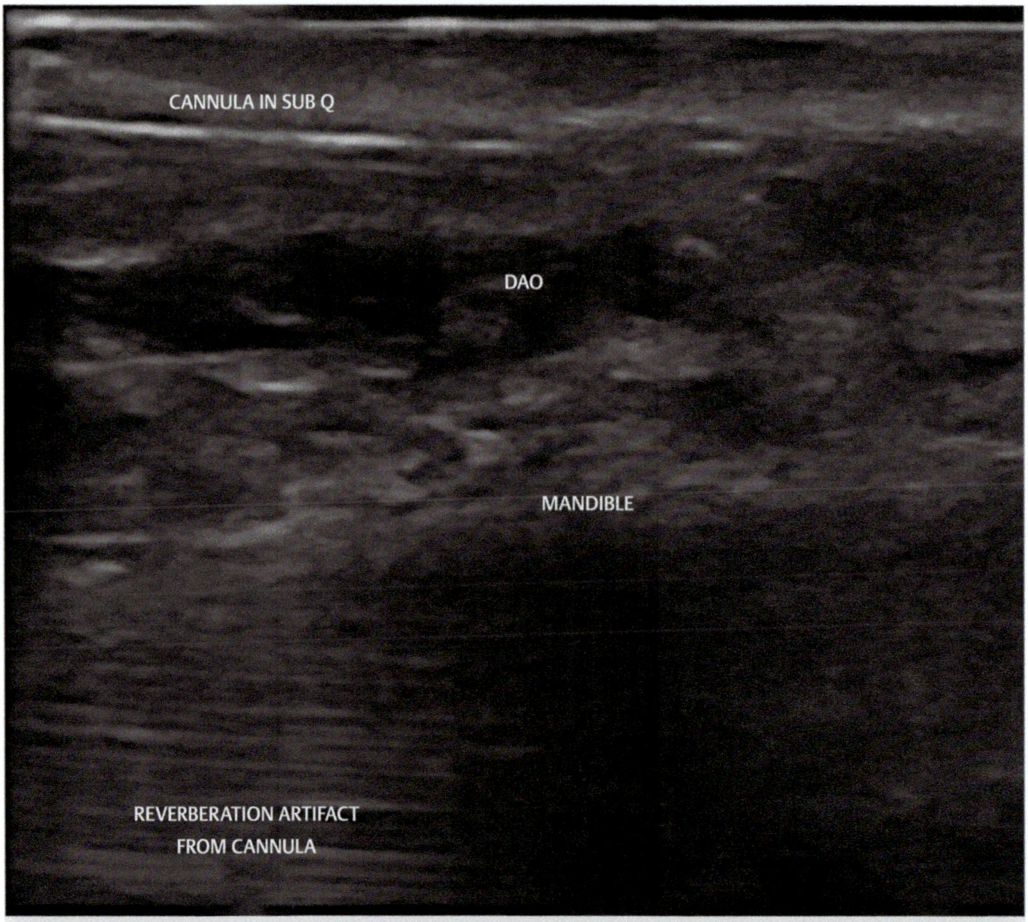

Fig. 4.26 Image obtained using a 20-MHz handheld probe. A cannula is placed between the depressor angulari oris (DAO) muscle and the dermis to subcise the labiomandibular ligament, which arises from the DAO and attaches to skin. This releases the ligament and improves the marionette depression. Reverberation artifact is caused by the sound wave reverberating within the lumen of the cannula and can be used to help identify where the needle/cannula is during guided injections.

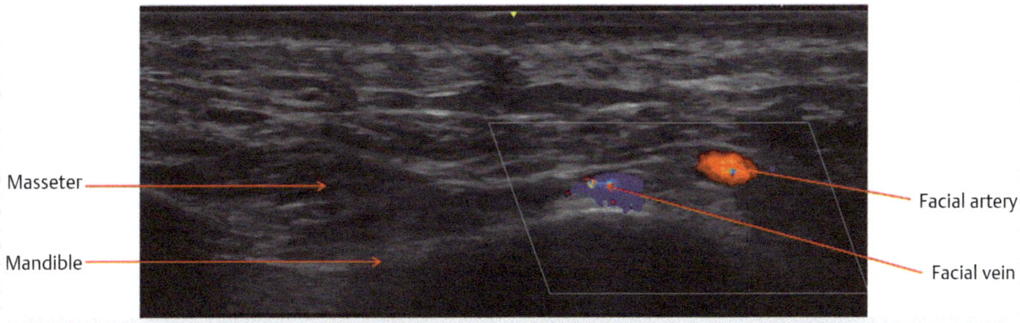

Fig. 4.27 Image obtained using an 20-MHz probe in horizontal position along the right mandibular border using color Doppler mode. The relationship of the facial artery (red) and facial vein (blue) in the antegonial notch. The vein is posterior to the artery in this image of the right lower face. Care must be exercised when visualizing the facial vein to apply minimal pressure with the probe, and it is advised to use an offset with abundance of gel when imaging.

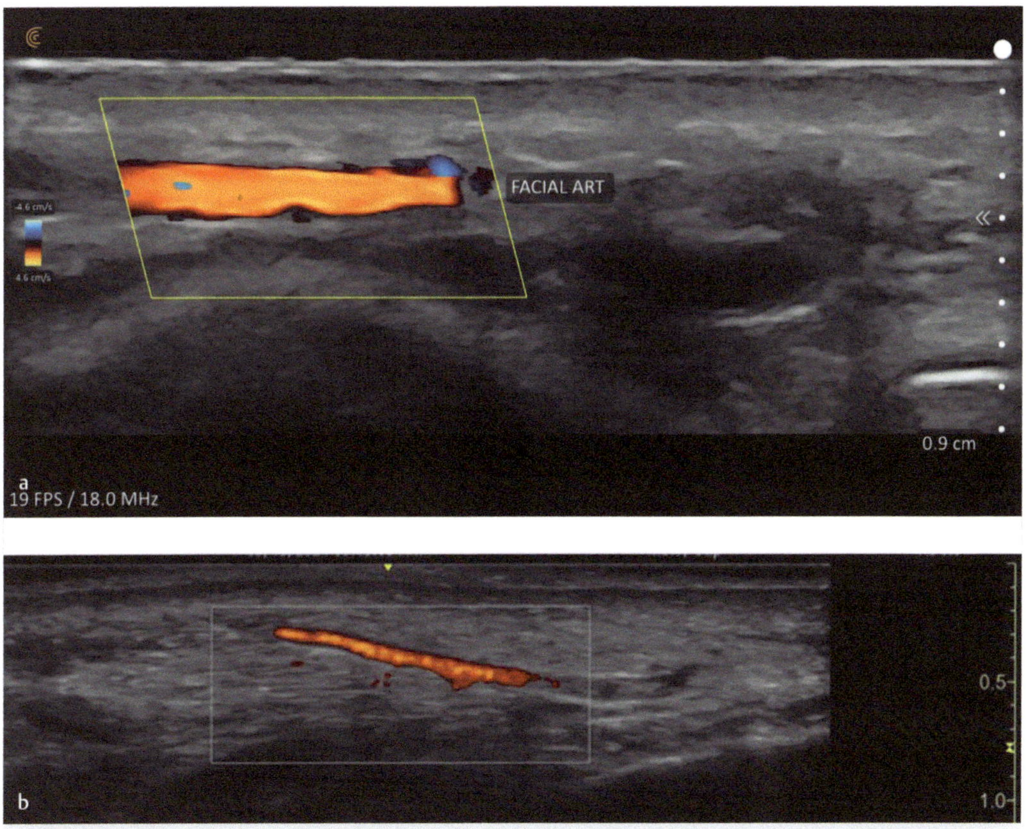

Fig. 4.28 (**a**) Image obtained using a 20-MHz handheld probe in vertical position, color Doppler. This image shows the facial artery traveling superiorly from the antegonial notch toward the oral commissure. The artery travels in the superficial musculoaponeurotic system (SMAS) layer in this area and is typically 4 to 5 mm deep. This is a high-velocity artery so velocity scale must be adjusted upward to avoid aliasing. The artery can be very tortuous in this area and capturing the entire length of the artery is difficult in one image. (**b**) Image obtained with a 20-MHz probe aligned with the nasolabial fold. Note that the depth of the angular artery is variable and becomes more superficial as it goes superiorly in this patient. It is at risk during nasolabial fold injections, particularly using needles, for a vascular occlusion.

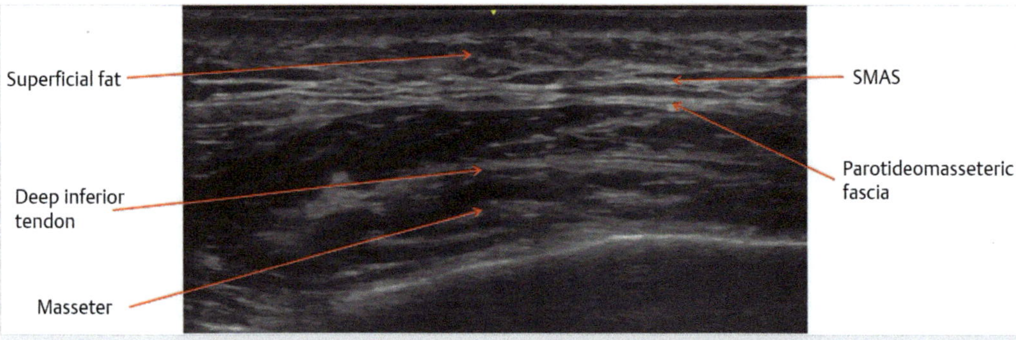

Fig. 4.29 Image obtained with a 20-MHz probe in horizontal orientation mid-jawline. The deep inferior tendon (DIT) divides the masseter into a superficial and deep component. It has been described that the masseter needs to be injected in both layers (above and below the DIT) to prevent the paradoxical bulging of the masseter after neurotoxin placement. It is both authors (SF and CS) recommendation to place filler above the SMAS when contouring the jawline with filler. Deep injections onto periosteum diffuse throughout the masseter over time and blunt the effect of the injection.

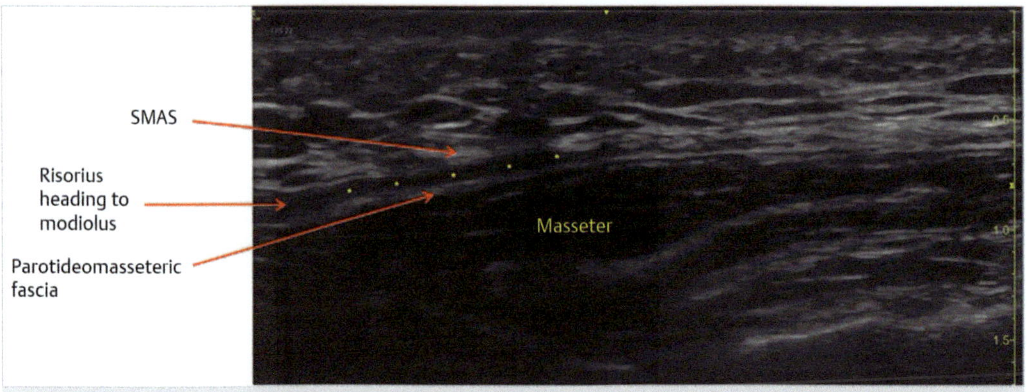

Fig. 4.30 The image is of a 20-MHz probe in a horizontal position at level of oral commissure. The risorius muscle arises from the anterior superficial surface of the parotideomasseteric fascia and extends anterior to insert into the modiolus. Its action is to widen the mouth, particularly during smiling. The importance of the risorius is that it can be inadvertently weakened during neurotoxin injections into the masseter. To avoid risorius during masseter injections, the author (SW) recommends injecting below a line drawn from the oral commissure to the ear lobe and posterior to the anterior border of the masseter (by palpation) by 1 cm.

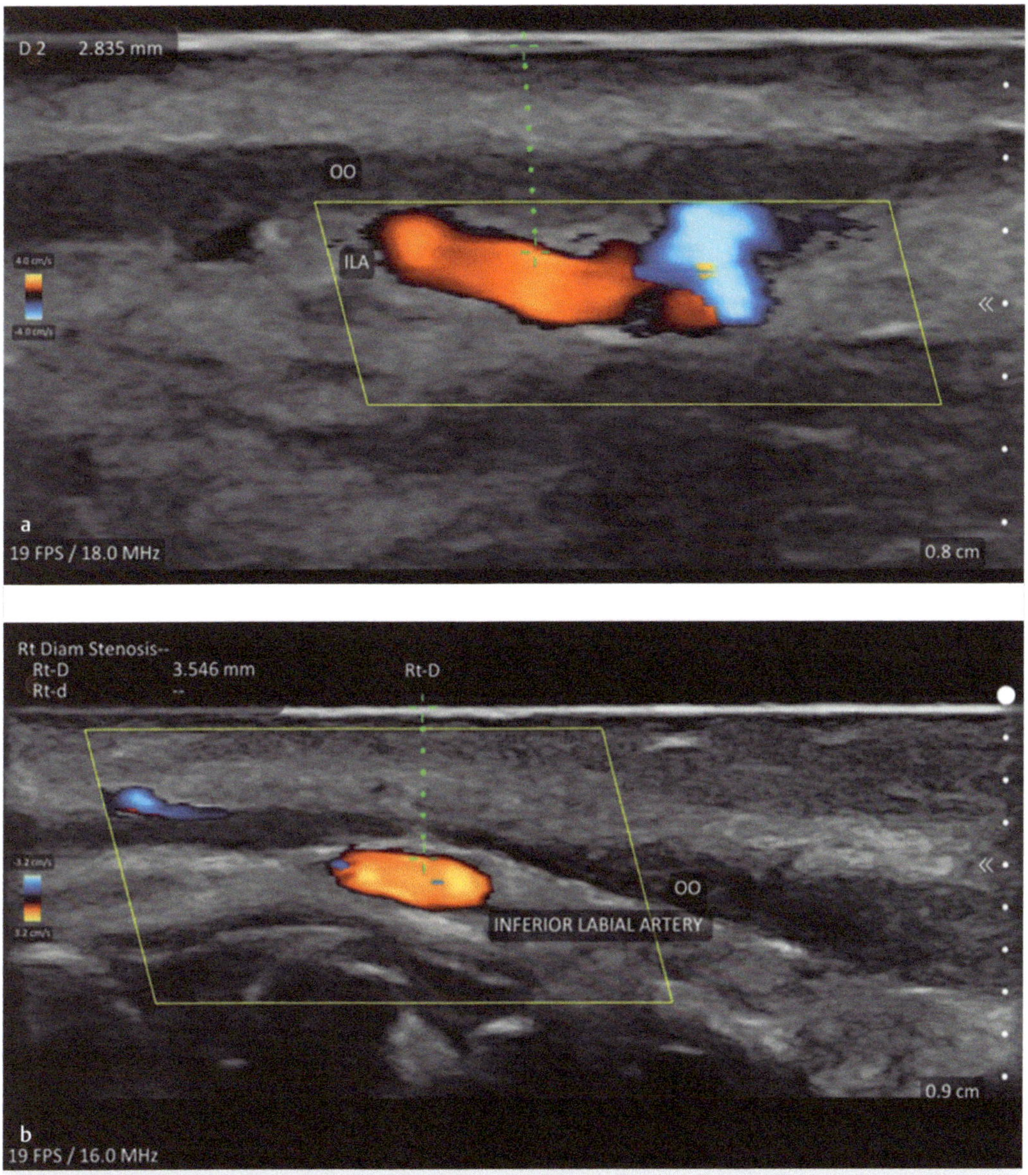

Fig. 4.31 **(a, b)** Image obtained using a 20-MHz handheld probe. The inferior labial artery (ILA) is shown deep to the orbicularis oris (OO) muscle in its typical location. The tortuous nature of the artery is common and is seen in this image with both red and blue flow of the vessel. Higher velocity scales need to be used because this is a high-flow vessel. Depth is typically about 3 mm. The lower image shows a component of the ILA lying superficial to the OO muscle.

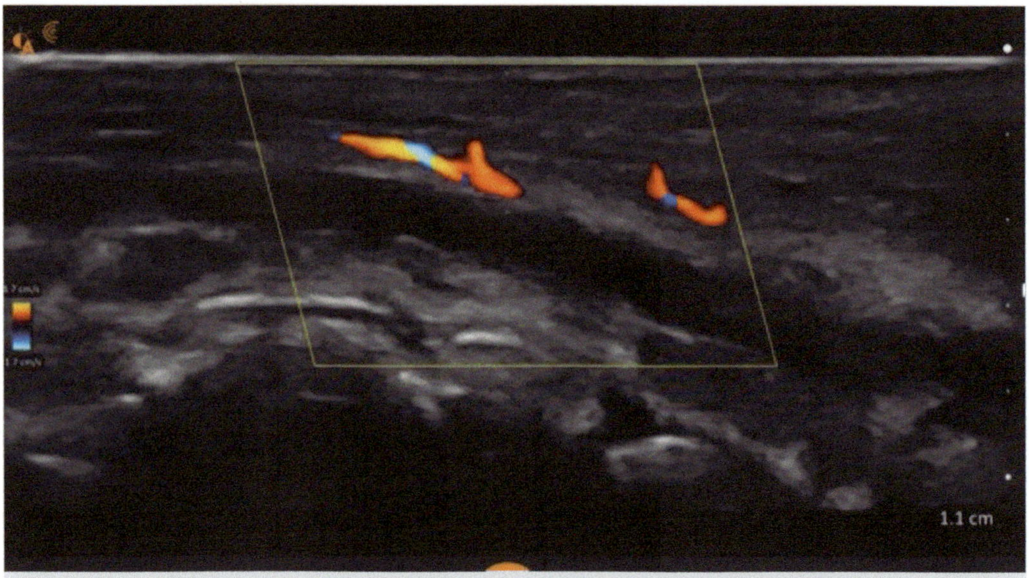

Fig. 4.32 Image obtained using a 20-MHz handheld probe in horizontal position. The inferior labial artery is seen lying superficial to the orbicularis oris muscle. This variant occurs at the rate of 2% and is at risk for occlusion.

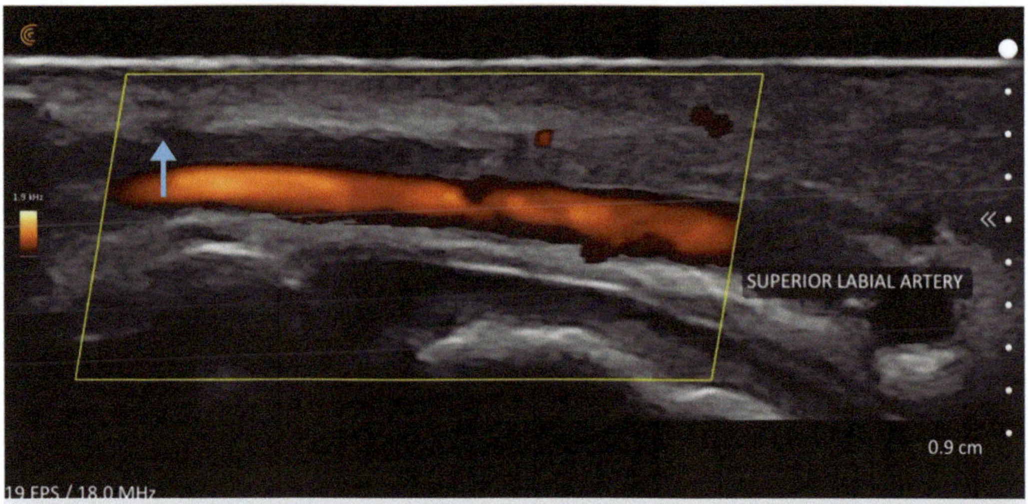

Fig. 4.33 Image obtained using a 20-MHz handheld probe using power Doppler mode. The superior labial artery (SLA) is typically seen deep to the orbicularis oris muscle (blue arrow). When compared to the inferior labial artery, the SLA is less tortuous.

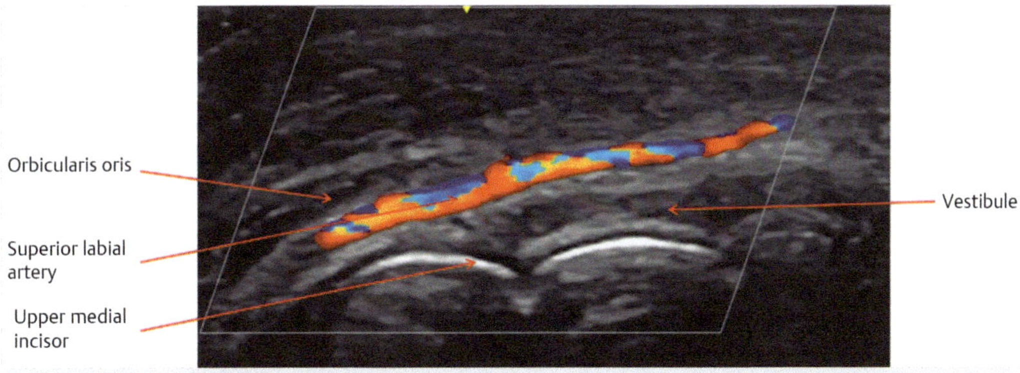

Fig. 4.34 Image obtained using an 18-MHz probe horizontally on upper lip. Note this artery is below the orbicularis oris. Vestibule lies just superficial to teeth.

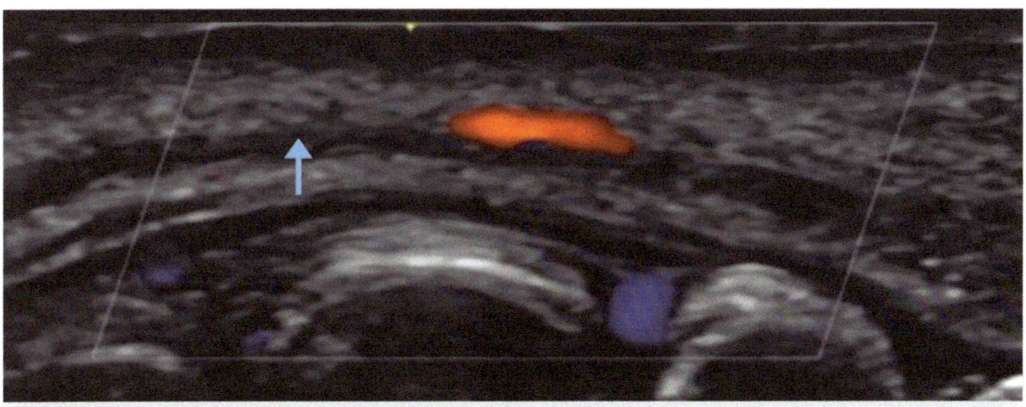

Fig. 4.35 Image obtained using an 18-MHz probe. The superior labial artery (SLA) is seen running superficial to the orbicularis oris muscle (blue arrow). This patient suffered a previous vascular occlusion when she had lip injections. A superficial SLA is probably a more common variant found in patients who have had lip vascular occlusions.

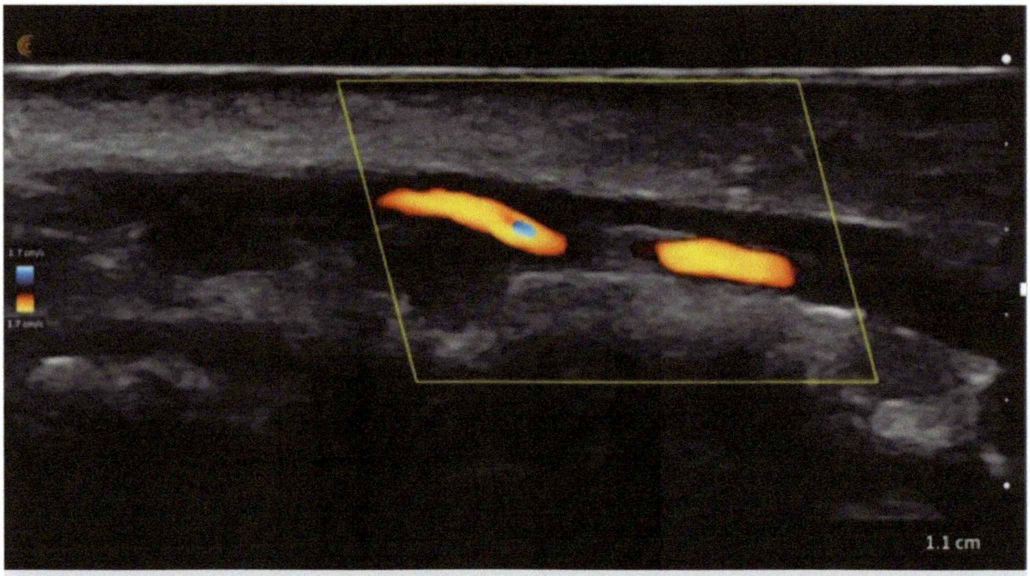

Fig. 4.36 Image obtained using a 20-MHz handheld probe in horizontal position. The superior labial artery is seen deep to the orbicularis oris muscle and within the same muscle. This variant occurs at a frequency of 24.14% according to Lee Walker's data.

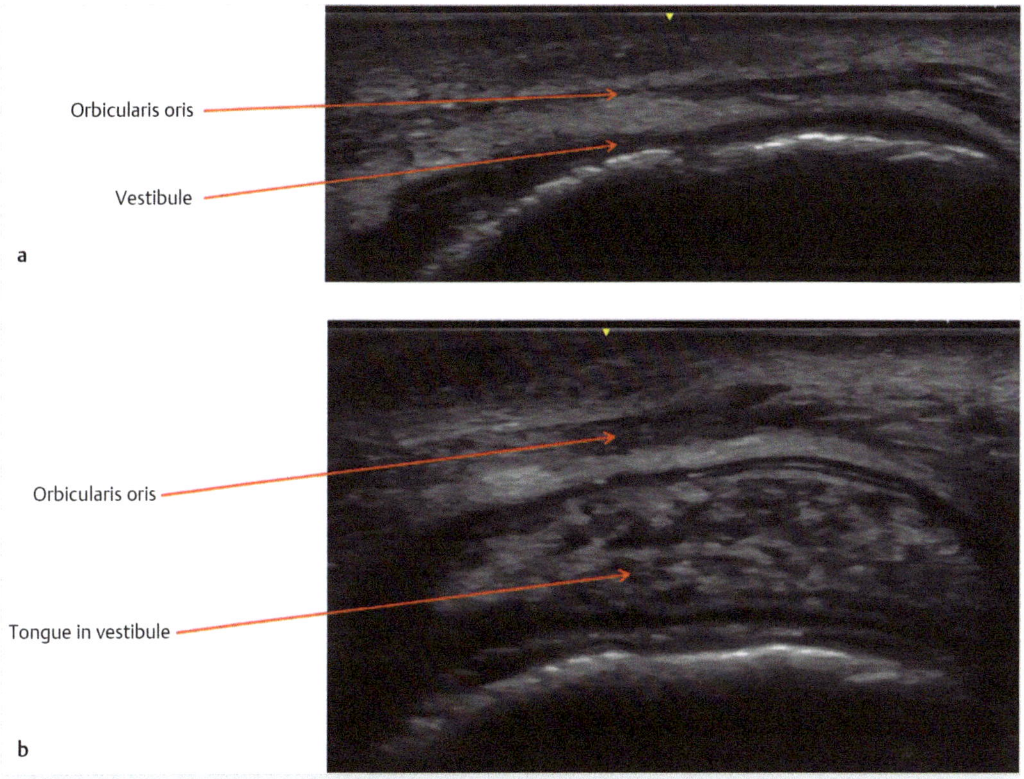

Fig. 4.37 (**a, b**) Images obtained using a 20-MHz probe horizontally on the upper lip. The anechoic vestibule is often confused with the orbicularis oris muscle but can be discerned from that by having the patient place their tongue between their teeth and lip.

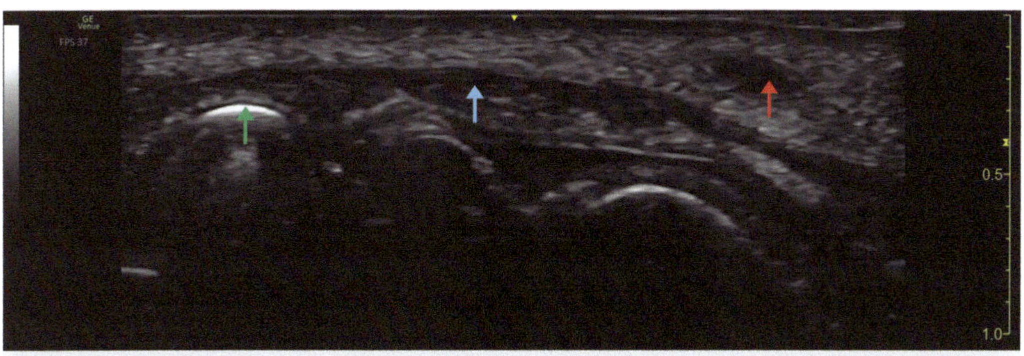

Fig. 4.38 Image obtained using an 18-MHz probe in horizontal position. This image shows the upper lip anatomy. Orbicularis oris muscle is anechoic/hypoechoic (blue arrow). Superficial fat pad is seen to contain a pocket of hyaluronic acid (HA) filler (red arrow). Teeth (green arrow) are hyperechoic and posterior to orbicularis oris muscle.

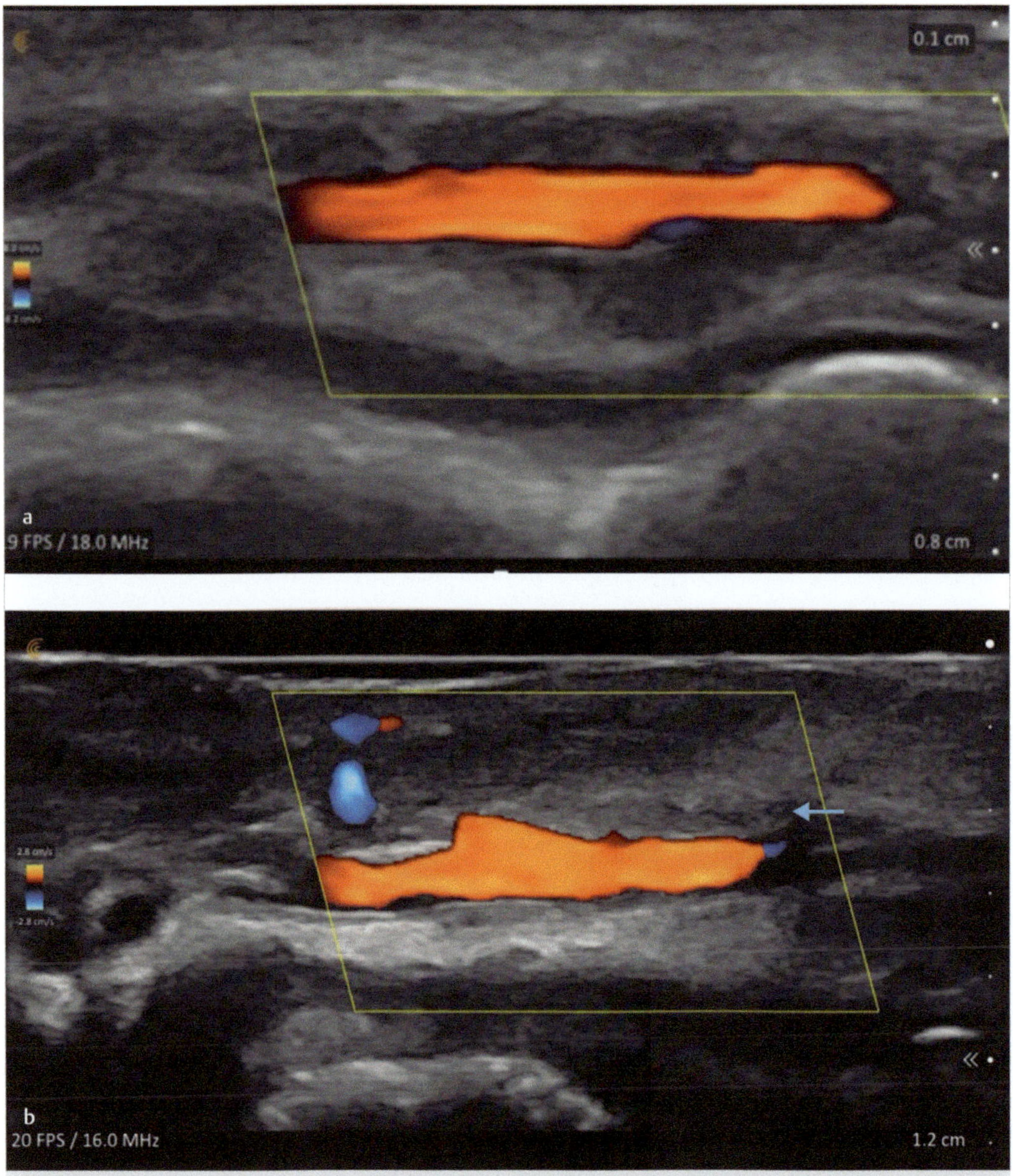

Fig. 4.39 (**a, b**) Image obtained using a 20-MHz handheld probe in horizontal position. The superior labial artery (SLA) can be seen sending off a philtral artery branch which becomes more superficial as it heads superiorly. Its typical depth is 2 mm and must be taken into consideration during injections in this area. Orbicularis oris muscle (blue arrow) is seen superficial to the SLA.

Suggested Readings

Bae JH, Choi DY, Lee JG, Seo KK, Tansatit T, Kim HJ. The risorius muscle: anatomic considerations with reference to botulinum neurotoxin injection for masseteric hypertrophy. Dermatol Surg. 2014; 40(12):1334–1339

Bhingardeo A. Accessory parotid gland and it's clinical significance. MedPulse International Journal of Anatomy. December 2020; 16(3):18-20

Cotofana S, Fratila AA, Schenck TL, Redka-Swoboda W, Zilinsky I, Pavicic T. The anatomy of the aging face: a review. Facial Plast Surg. 2016; 32(3):253–260

Cotofana S, Hong WJ, Horne J, et al. Intralabial lip compartments and their potential clinical relevance. Plast Reconstr Surg. 2023

Crouzet C, Fournier H, Papon X, Hentati N, Cronier P, Mercier P. Anatomy of the arterial vascularization of the lips. Surg Radiol Anat. 1998; 20(4):273–278

Edizer M, Mağden O, Tayfur V, Kiray A, Ergür I, Atabey A. Arterial anatomy of the lower lip: a cadaveric study. Plast Reconstr Surg. 2003; 111(7):2176–2181

Faizal B, Chandran MP. Pneumoparotitis. Amrita Journal of Medicine. 2012; 8(2):1–44. Archived from the original (PDF) on 2015-12-11

Ferreira-Pileggi BC, Freire AR, Botacin PR, Prado FB, Rossi AC. A Different Pattern of Arrangement of the Risorius Muscle Fibers: A Case Report. Cureus. 2022 Mar 7;14(3):e22922

Frommer J. The human accessory parotid gland: its incidence, nature, and significance. Oral Surg Oral Med Oral Pathol. 1977; 43(5):671–676

Furukawa M, Mathes DW, Anzai Y. Evaluation of the facial artery on computed tomographic angiography using 64-slice multidetector computed tomography: implications for facial reconstruction in plastic surgery. Plast Reconstr Surg. 2013; 131(3):526–535

Huettner F, Rueda S, Ozturk CN, et al. The relationship of the marginal mandibular nerve to the mandibular osseocutaneous ligament and lesser ligaments of the lower face. Aesthet Surg J. 2015; 35(2):111–120

Lamb J, Surek C. Facial Volumization: An Anatomic Approach. 1st ed. New York: NY: Thieme Medical Publishers; 2017

Lee HJ, Kang IW, Seo KK, et al. The anatomical basis of paradoxical masseteric bulging after botulinum neurotoxin Type A injection. Toxins (Basel). 2016; 9(1):14

Lee SH, Gil YC, Choi YJ, Tansatit T, Kim HJ, Hu KS. Topographic anatomy of the superior labial artery for dermal filler injection. Plast Reconstr Surg. 2015; 135(2):445–450

Loukas M, Hullett J, Louis RG, Jr, et al. A detailed observation of variations of the facial artery, with emphasis on the superior labial artery. Surg Radiol Anat. 2006; 28(3):316–324

Mendelson BC, Freeman ME, Wu W, Huggins RJ. Surgical anatomy of the lower face: the premasseter space, the jowl, and the labiomandibular fold. Aesthetic Plast Surg. 2008; 32(2):185–195

Nakajima H, Imanishi N, Aiso S. Facial artery in the upper lip and nose: anatomy and a clinical application. Plast Reconstr Surg. 2002; 109(3):855–861, discussion 862–863

Pinar YA, Bilge O, Govsa F. Anatomic study of the blood supply of perioral region. Clin Anat. 2005; 18(5):330–339

Prativadi R, Dahiya N, Kamaya A, Bhatt S. Chapter 5 Ultrasound Characteristics of Benign vs Malignant Cervical Lymph Nodes, Seminars in Ultrasound, CT and MRI. 2017: 38(5): 506-515

Rosengaus-Leizgold F, Jasso-Ramírez E, Sicilia NC. The Happy Face treatment: an anatomical-based technique for the correction of marionette lines and the oral commissures. J Drugs Dermatol. 2018; 17(11):1226–1228

Schelke L, Schoonen T, Velthuis PJ. Filler injections in the pre-auricular space: Be aware of the parotid gland. J Cosmet Dermatol. 2023; 22 (1):173–176

Surek C. "Facial Anatomy for Filler Injection: The Superficial Musculoaponeurotic System (SMAS) is Not Just for Facelifting" Clinics in Plastic Surgery. Editors Zins, Charafeddine. Philadelphia, PA. Elsevier

Surek CC, Guisantes E, Schnarr K, Jelks G, Beut J. "No-touch" technique for lip enhancement. Plast Reconstr Surg. 2016; 138(4): 603e–613e

Tansatit T, Apinuntrum P, Phetudom T. A typical pattern of the labial arteries with implication for lip augmentation with injectable fillers. Aesthetic Plast Surg. 2014; 38(6):1083–1089

Walker, L., Cetto, R. Bruke, T. Facial Ageing and Injection Anatomy: A Compendium of Evidenced Based Principles. 2021. UK Book Publishing

2014 by the American Society for Dermatologic Surgery, Inc. Published by Lippincott Williams & Wilkins. ISSN: 1076–0512. Dermatol Surg 2014;40:1334–1339.

Index

Note: Page numbers set **bold** or *italic* indicate headings or figures, respectively.